Hatha Yoga Practice

Disciple against Wall

Shanti Nathini

(Maria Nikolaeva)

First Russian Edition:

Ritambhara Publishing House (Moscow, 2005)

Demonstration of Asanas:

Shanti Nathini, Surinder Singh, Edgar Ortize, Michael Jekel

Photography: Maria Nikolaeva, Mikhail Tzelman

Correction: Tatiana Morozova

Cover Design: Oleg Kosarev

ISBN 1-4196-6105-1

To order additional copies, please contact us.
BookSurge Publishing
www.booksurge.com
1-866-308-6235
orders@booksurge.com

Hatha Yoga Practice
Disciple against Wall

Shanti Nathini

(Maria Nikolaeva)

BookSurge Publishing
2007

Hatha Yoga Practice

Disciple against Wall

Preface.
Hatha Yoga Schools in Russia

Contemporary 'Yoga' is equal to 'asana' for many westerners, which don't discriminate between 'Yoga' and 'Hatha Yoga' and treat 'meditation' as a separate subject. Modern Hatha Yoga is not the same everywhere; there are a lot of different schools based on several major traditions. Each school of Hatha Yoga finds the way for development in India and abroad including Russia. Practice of Yoga was prohibited in Soviet Union, though some people could learn asanas illegally, but during the last twenty years Yoga has been spreading all over the Russia very fast. Except of some articles on Yoga as a physical culture published in Soviet period, originally Yoga appeared in Russia thanks to self-developed Yoga-masters who learned asanas by themselves from books. They became first Yoga-teachers and their disciples taught Yoga in many cities like Moscow, Petersburg etc. As a result when the genuine Indian tradition came to Russia it found a paved way for itself but at the same time it was required to satisfy the special needs of Russian mentality, which was unusual for Indian yogis. In an extremely difficult period of political and economic change in the motherland serious character of Russians forced them to apply the highest results in asana-practice and the deepest studying of Yoga-philosophy, trying to discover the truest sense of human life. After reading the next pages Dr. Frawley wrote to me: 'I do hope that the Russian Yoga goes more deeply into the greater Yoga tradition and the great spiritual gurus of Yoga than what is happening in the USA'.

That is why you should not be surprised that in a very short historical period in Russia a lot of Yoga-centers were established, many professional Yoga-teachers appeared among Russians, and Yoga have already become the important part of daily life for the majority of educated people and students of institutes. Book-shops are full of translated literature on different Yoga-traditions, and some years ago first Russian Yoga Magazine started to be published four times a year. Also even ordinary people can practice simple Yoga in any fitness-club, where the main aim is the restoration of health and emotional stability after a hard working day. During the recent years Yoga has become a special subject of studying in philosophical departments of state universities, and students are allowed to maintain a diploma-work in Yoga as a science. Russian indologists translated from Sanskrit into Russian many classical texts on Yoga such as *'Yoga Sutras'*, *'Bhagavad-Gita'*, *'Yoga Upanishads'*, *'Hatha Yoga Pradipika'* etc., and now anybody can read these books in his mother tongue. Definitely Yoga in Russia is the vast area for scientific research, and in this article we'll try to reflect on the destiny of the most famous Indian Yoga-schools after their contact with distinctive Russian culture.

2

Iyengar Yoga in Russia

It is well-known that Yoga became widely popular in Western countries after the famous yogacharya B.K.S. Iyengar visited Europe in the middle of XX century, and according to general opinion till the present time Iyengar Yoga is the most attractive stile of practice for people in the entire world. Certainly Russia didn't become an exception: B.K.S. Iyengar came to Moscow at the end of October in 1989 to participate in the First Russian Yoga Conference, and he stayed there for about ten days. Obviously practical teaching was the most important part of his work, including two mega-classes for the whole crowd of concerned people. First of all yogacharya asked them to remove socks and denude knees, but just after Soviet period it was completely unusual and even such simple action made a splash. All people tried to perform asanas with great enthusiasm, and of course they asked many very different questions. However there were too many new terms in teacher's answers, and interpreting was not good enough for proper understanding of direct sense. Anyway, Iyengar's visit produced inexhaustible inspiration for self-practice, and people continued to learn Iyengar Yoga themselves at home during the next several years.

In 1992 B.K.S. Iyengar gave an official permission to establish the first Yoga center in Russia, and in spite of some problems Moscow Iyengar Yoga Center was opened just one year later. Now, after almost 15 years full of innumerable and indescribable difficulties and advances this center has several Yoga-halls in the city and about twenty professional Yoga-teachers. It's difficult to count, but it's possible that more than several thousand people became permanent students of Iyengar Yoga and it's not the final result: every day the administrators answer endless phone-calls. New Iyengar Yoga centers were established in Petersburg and other Russian cities, and they are developing successfully, as well as some groups in Ukraine and Moldova. The first Russian translation of the book *'Light on Yoga'* by B.K.S. Iyengar appeared in 1993 and was reprinted many times though later all other books by the same author were published in Russian. Also you can find alternative editions on Iyengar Yoga, for instance this my book is dedicated to technical explanation how to master asanas with the support of wall, basically according to main principles of using props intrinsic to Iyengar Yoga. But it's necessary to emphasize that I don't follow them strictly. It's just an example, because there is a choice in literature on this topic.

Talking of the historical development of Iyengar Yoga in Russia it's necessary to notice the peculiar role of Faek Beria, the favorite disciple of B.K.S. Iyengar and the director of Paris Iyengar Yoga Center. First he went to Moscow from France in 1989 specifically to accompany his teacher, but Iyengar himself asked him to visit Russia from time to time and teach Yoga there. Faek Beria accepted the responsibility and for many years he became a guardian of Iyengar Yoga in Russia and the very favorite Yoga teacher. Just one month after the First Russian Yoga Conference he came back to Moscow to give some classes and support the interested people, who couldn't imagine their life without Yoga. In 1990 Faek Beria came to Moscow again but except of a common class he took part in a TV-program for popularization of Iyengar Yoga in the entire Russia. Next time he visited Petersburg, and just one year later there was a permanent group of Yoga-practitioners which established new Petersburg Iyengar Yoga Center. Faek Beria's seminars still attract a lot of Russian people almost every year. As a whole, you can see a good example of indirect way, by which sometimes Yoga goes from India through Europe to Russia.

Ashtanga Vinyasa Yoga in Russia

Though Iyengar Yoga is without doubt recognized in Russia, we should emphasize that Ashtanga Vinyasa Yoga is much more popular. The keeper of this Hatha Yoga style is Pattabhi Jois from Mysore, who is respected by practitioners, however Ashtanga Vinyasa Yoga is taught by Russian Yoga-teachers in a different way. Basically the vinyasa (dynamic sequence of asanas) is accepted as a principle but the order of asanas complies with the so-called 'Free Flow', and each class is different from another one. In Moscow and Petersburg every beginner can choose one of such Yoga-teachers, who don't claim that they teach Ashtanga Vinyasa Yoga, though their stile is very similar to this type of practice. Still there aren't any Russian Yoga-teachers certificated by Pattabhi Jois himself, but it seems normal since the rules of the examinations are very exact including the request to come to South India for one month in the year during three years or longer. Of course, it's not a simple task for Russians. At the same time you can find in Russia a few places where people practice classical Ashtanga Vinyasa Yoga in groups. At least occasionally they give special lessons on First Sequence of asanas and anybody can receive direct experience of Ashtanga Vinyasa Yoga as such.

The Ashtanga Yoga Center is the most valid Russian organization where you can study traditional Ashtanga Vinyasa Yoga. It has branches both in Moscow and Petersburg and it is recognized by International Yoga Federation. In recent years many Yoga-teachers from this center have visited Mysore, practiced with Pattabhi Jois himself, and then they give daily classes separately for beginners and advanced practitioners. In addition they organize short intensive seminars on classical Ashtanga Vinyasa Yoga not only in Russia but also in India: for instance, regular seminar will be held by Mikhail Konstantinov, the leader of Moscow Ashtanga Yoga Center, in Goa, where also Russian Yoga Center exists permanently. But other Yoga styles are also acceptable in the center, and Ashtanga Vinyasa Yoga doesn't contradict to other noble traditions. For example, Bal Mukund Singh, the most famous disciple of Sri Dhirendra Brahmachari, was invited to Russia two years ago, and he held successful workshops both in Moscow and Petersburg.

The main principle of Ashtanga Vinyasa Yoga reads as follows: 99% practice + 1% theory. Pattabhi Jois has written three books only. The most important of his treatises *'Yoga Mala'* was translated into Russian long time ago and published in the Ukraine. Besides people can find the description of this style in my own book *'Hatha Yoga Practice: Disciple among Teachers',* published in Petersburg and reprinted in Moscow. In my work a separate chapter was dedicated to my own experience in Ashtanga Vinyasa Yoga, received in Mysore with two other famous teachers B.N.S. Iyengar and V. Sheshadri. In the supplement you can see the First Sequence of Ashtanga Vinyasa Yoga in pictures, which contains almost one hundred asanas. For future Ritambhara Publishing House, attached to Moscow Ashtanga Yoga Center, is preparing for publishing the first Russian translation of book *'Ashtanga Yoga'* written by a western Yoga-teacher Jon Scott. Some new articles on Ashtanga Vinyasa Yoga appear periodically in Russian Yoga Magazine under the editorship of Mikhail Konstantinov, and the September, 2005 issue was dedicated to 90-th anniversary of Pattabhi Jois as the holder of traditional Ashtanga Vinyasa Yoga, who continues to teach and inspire disciples by his own example of Yoga-life. Mikhail Konstantinov, who is also a director of Ashtanga Yoga Centre, has been recognized as the first Russian certified Yoga teacher of this style. For sure, Ashtanga Vinyasa Yoga will become more and more popular in Russia.

Other Yoga Schools in Russia

Certainly all other schools of Hatha Yoga are well-known in Russia and gradually they find their followers, although they don't become so popular as Iyengar Yoga and Ashtanga Vinyasa Yoga. As you know, both these styles are raised to Sri Krishnamacharya, who was the guru of both B.K.S. Iyengar and Pattabhi Jois. Nevertheless he made his own son the successor and holder of his main tradition, and until now T.K.V. Desikachar is teaching Vini Yoga in Chennai. But this style didn't spread too vast neither in India nor abroad. It is not famous in Russia also: only the Ukrainian master Andrey Lappa completed a full course of education in Krishnamacharya Yoga Mandiram under the guidance of Desikachar himself, but he integrated this knowledge into his own system and he never teaches Vini Yoga as such. Despite the failure of this branch, Russian yogis respect Sri Krishnamacharya as one of the main staffs of contemporary Hatha Yoga. Evidently his fame owes its existence to the fact that Sri Krishnamacharya studied philosophy in Benares University during as many as ten years. In his case the development of intelligence became the base for reconstruction of ancient yogic tradition and its adaptation to modern society.

Another great yogacharya of XX Century Swami Sivananda Saraswati also became a source of several Hatha-yogic schools, and his teaching got interesting ways of development in Russia. As you know, he established the Divine Life

Society in Rishikesh, and his disciple's activity created the big-gest net of Sivananda-ashrams in the entire world, both in India and many Western countries. Of course, Sivananda Yoga is well-known to Russians from books, and yet there is no Yoga center where beginner could study only this style of practice, without any mixing with other traditions. It is the monastic char-acter of this school that may be the reason for that, since Swami Sivananda was a sannyasin, but it's almost impossible to found ashrams resembling Indian tradition in Russia. At the same time many Yoga-teachers accept the basic principles of Sivananda Yoga for holding classes in some fitness-clubs, where people need relaxation and restoration of emotional stability. The simi-lar destiny overtook the teaching of Bihar School of Yoga, founded by Swami Satyananda Saraswati, the most famous disciple of Swami Sivananda Saraswati. Everybody in Russia knows such his techniques as Yoga Nidra, Swara Yoga etc, and Yoga-teachers put them into practice but still nobody teaches Satyananda Yoga systematically.

We could continue this overview with long enumeration of Indian yogacharyas who influenced the development of Russian Yoga in a varying degree at his personal visit or just owing to his books. Generally it can be said without exaggeration that Rus-sian practitioners aspire to master Yoga under auspices of dif-ferent Yoga-teachers because they are interested to understand Yoga as such, without isolation inside of one and only school. Though you can find plenty of Yoga centers and Yoga-teachers in Russia today, even now some people study Yoga by themselves from books and on their own experience, trusting their own intuition and understanding. Original yogis who live in small towns find essential support visiting seminars in the closest cities, where they are able to participate. Russian Yoga-teachers like to organize short intensive seminars with the filled daily program. Fruitful meetings with Indian yogacharyas also become part and parcel in Russian yogi's lives, and international contacts can easily happen in the territory of their own country as well as in the motherland of Yoga itself. Progressively Russian practitioners believe that Yoga-practice is the best way to the ultimate Self-realization.

Introduction.
Metaphorical 'Dead End'

'Wall' seems to be a metaphorical dead end on the spiritual way; however, we can interpret this metaphor literally. When a disciple is forced to interact with himself, he finds himself in front of a blind wall without his teacher, besides the wall becomes the dependable means for reflection. Actually, there is nobody outside you, if your Self is all-inclusive. But while you don't encounter the barrier, you generally perceive all to be outdoors, except yourself. Whenever you fall into a really deadlock condition, in the first instance you face yourself in the concrete. In the full glare into your depth an inner space arises inside and starts to expand inexorably, while the wall appears to be somewhere beneath, scarcely distinguishable from spiritual level.

Extremity is similar to inspiration; and after a brief irresolution you ask an inevitable question: how to work with the wall which blocked your path? Hatha Yoga is profoundly symbolical like any practice rooted in mystical Tantrism. In order to get outside of 'the wall' in the general sense, you should approach a real wall. And as a simplest solution you can practice Yoga 'with the support of a wall'. Nevertheless the situation is not completed in the same way, since the wall extricates from a block to vertical, establish new dimension for life and practice. The first wall access is destined mainly for beginners, but with the further development of volume in the practice the wall offers plenty opportunities for advanced students. The wall is accustomed and becomes a small part of the life-structure, and then you are able to move it on your own will, disposing it at any angle.

At the very beginning the wall is perceived as an obstacle, but actually it becomes a turning point in your practice, permission to be directed upwards, to advance your mastery and personal energy. The wall is a great teacher, for every possible enlightenment starts from the proper work of your body. This body includes everything. So, if you know your own body 'through and through' and you are able to control it, then there is nothing that does not correspond to your conscious decisions. Contemporary situation redoubles together with evolving of Hatha Yoga practice, which I denominated in one of my previous books as 'disciple among teachers'. Everything is equal to nothing; and many of the Yoga-instructors are not different from the wall, which recovers your inner guru. But still, don't worship it; apply the wall forbearingly, since it is nothing more than an external sign or marker on the way up.

Acknowledgements

I'm grateful to Swami Dharmananda (International Himalayan Vishwaguru Yoga University, India) for attention to my research and kindly support, and Russian Yoga-teacher Mikhail Konstantinov, the director of Ashtanga Yoga Centre and chief editor of Ritambhara Publishing House, for the original edition of this book in Moscow. My special acknowledgement is to Dr. David Frawley (Pandit Vamadeva Shastri), director of American Institute of Vedic Studies, for his reference on English manuscript and some comments from his side which are fundamental for my other books.

Also I express my gratitude to Yoga teacher Surinder Singh (India) and practitioners Edgar Ortiz (Costa Rica) and Michael Jekel (Germany), who demonstrated asanas for exposure; to all Iyengar Yoga teachers, who pointed out working techniques with support of wall (though I don't follow them strictly) and Yoga instructors of other styles for specification of aspects; as well to Yoga practitioners who helped to make pictures: Mikhail Tzelman (USA) and Yasue Murata (Japan). My thanks are due to Tatiana Morozova, the Yoga teacher and translator, for English manuscript correction, and to Oleg Kosarev, the programmer, for the cover artwork design.

Part I.
Theory: Entrance to Vertical

The wall is a sort of vertical 'landing-strip', where you gather speed of Self-realization. Interaction with the wall acts as a psychological workshop in a greater measure, than mastering of physical form. However stop short of perversion: this is not Yoga with 'cold partner', but the practical way to become aware of your own body. First of all Hatha Yoga practice is the work with consciousness and energy, therefore you should not cherish illusions on importance of the body as such. Primarily the wall testifies physical disability in front of barrier, where you can understand and feel this disability. Any corporal-oriented training is intended to convert knowledge about your existence into experience of your objective reality. The question is how you are living currently – on the flat or on several levels of being?

The common man scurries between coming and going horizontal energy flows, produced by their scrappy thoughts, absurd impulsions, disorderly actions caused by other similar people. In the chaos he tries to pave wandering way to nowhere or just beyond the horizon on the same level of consciousness, merely marking the limit of perception. Do you embrace highest sky overhead and deepest earth underfoot? This question is far from lyrical. The development of energy structure supposes the vertical orientation of consciousness. More simply, in awaked state the bodily axis is positioned directly, and it consists from the links between conscious centers on different levels. In such a way Hatha Yogis work with charkas inside of Sushumna, while you can find alternative options for nurturance of realization in other traditions. But principally this is the vertical movement.

Volume Realization in Yoga Practice

Theoretically the wall sets up third-dimensional coordinates and forms 'volume awareness'. Usually Hatha Yoga practice takes place on horizontal floor only. You fail to get rid of habitual stream of consciousness even during whole two hours, since you continue to take action on the same level. As you know, visual environment depends on state of consciousness, and if you start thinking more 'sublime', then the former world disperses and a new world concentrates around. Instead of elevation you strive to imitate an instructor's posture, looking for other practitioners, and their shapes provoke a lot of extraneous whirls in mind. You are irreparably smeared-out 'floor screen', and there's nothing to be done but to slide on surface, as if you would be like shadow, which is unable to observe improvement.

Access to the wall adds instantly a chance to correlate with vertical surface, especially when you stay face to face with it. You discover third coordinate axis that is the height, which hitherto was present somewhere in under-self only, but you never match up this line consciously. Nevertheless you always exist in the midst of vertical planes such as walls, trees, rocks etc.; just you constantly project them under your feet and skillfully skirt their imagery. Intentional inclusion of asanas 'on the wall' into practice is not so much artificial means, as return to native habitat of human being. Appearance of summit and bottom out of eyeshot is similar to elementary enlightenment, but as you know any enlightenment is never ultimate. Just you start understanding the principle of gradual extension of consciousness, and then you learn to gain advantage in self-development.

As a preliminary let us mention a kind of such a curious 'flash' at runtime of headstand, which was described with a real yogic humor by Essudian and Heich. The result of regular Shirshasana practice looks like a miracle. Following lingering persuasion 'neurotic' or 'victim technocratic society' starts performing Shirshasana incredulously and indifferent. At the first attempt he doesn't succeed to stand on his head, and feet seem to adhere to floor area, but he feels some flush of freshness. Next day he tries again, *first at the wall,* and now he is able to remove feet from the floor, although he cannot straighten legs upwards. Giving over futile attempts he gets on his feet again with wonderful sense… Then he laughs! On the following day it is obtained a shade better. Finishing Yoga practice he sits in the armchair and suddenly can reads without any glasses; toward the evening he notes dissolution of usual singing in the ears;

and the next morning he brings back to memory, that he forgot oneself in sleep without an accustomed dose of soporific drug…

It is the case, since the inversion restores the feeling of vertical axis, which is an 'identification post' for conscious centering. Debugged work of sensory organs and equability of nervous system directly depend on availability of inner 'column'. Balancing on his head for the first time with full attention, anybody concentrates an amorphous cloud of awareness to the vertical line. This is just the direction of thinking or transmitted radiation from top downward. But because he need to entrench himself in this abstraction, he starts embodying it into his own energetic structure. Of course everything starts from self-visualization not on the horizontal surface but along the vertical axis. Then this imagination commences to take shape of tuning work out vertical energetic channel, and further externalizes oneself into perfect coordination of formerly weakened connections between different parts of body.

It will be observed that Hatha Yoga masters give consideration to extensionality of the practice construction very rear in distinction from adepts of Tantra concerned with arising of Kundaliny. Mostly Hatha Yogis emphasize to create asana sequences, exploiting usual one-dimensional thinking, but almost not invoking capability for extension of consciousness. However there are several attempts, and for instance we quote the conception of Andrey Lappa. He tries to set up not only some sequences, but integral system, called 'multilevel algorithm of vinyasas' by him. Here 'vinyasa' means dynamical set that is the repetition of some asanas according to contra-posture principle in general, taking into account the compensating action. Application of this algorithm enables him to form Yantra or universal technological yogic diagram. More simply he puts into consciousness all asanas at once, in addition ordering them not on the surface only, but also according to level of complexity in terms of type of support.

Hierarchy of vinyasas is constructed as transition from simple to complex, from less effective to more effective. For example, if somebody is not able to perform hand-stand, then all inverted asanas are represented for him variations in headstand and shoulder-stand. Try as one would to combine accessible postures, while level of his ability will not be increased to the next-higher order, he will not pass on the next level of practice, where most of asanas are performed with support on the hands. Basic vinyasas operate for 'starting' and 'rotating' of psycho-energetic Mandala. Their powerful influence depends on some effects, especially on the next one. Inversion of head and spine in space influences basic subconscious 'fixations' to direction of gravitational field, therefore the intensity of energetic structure steps up.

This complex structure is completely and nobly presented in the book 'Yoga: Tradition of Union' by Andrey Lappa himself. But here it is necessary for us to note *vertical* and *volume* only.

Walls of House: Vastu of Yoga Shala

Walls confine some volume of space, which is used for Yoga-hall or house, where you spend most of your time. This well-defined volume is most commonly recognized as a territory, existing in planar dimension again. However we should give special attention to this limited space. Indeed in Hatha Yoga practice we develop sensibility, starting from the plain and un-equivocal perception of the body in all structural aspects but finishing with the very physical feeling of entire Universe. Emphatically there are some intermediate intelligible contents between these almost incommensurable quantities. This is a reason why such magic sciences as Chinese Feng Shui, Indian Vastu and many other types of geomantic knowledge were developed almost in all cultures from hoary antiquity.

Frequently Hatha Yoga practitioners are inclinable to neglect these rules. They are sure that alignment of body by itself influence environment, forcing it to tune with inner changing. Principally, they are right, but the only question at issue is the degree of force exertion. For instance, in order to remove calculus from kidney exclusively by energetic methods you will need to waste immeasurable more subtle energy, than in the case when you will take advantage of rougher remedy like herbs, massage etc. At the limit it is safe to say that only stupid person will light up a candle by force of his glance, if he has matches in hand. That is why yogis prohibit the demonstration of risen siddhi (supernatural power). It is equally true that Feng Shui and Vastu practice will be the 'least-cost' one from the viewpoint of your energy consumption, especially in an infant state. Better don't try to expand 'Procrustean bed' by powerful radiation.

Moreover rules of this sort are never mechanical, but these prescriptions require the development of sensibility also. In such a way learning Feng Shui and Vastu you continue Yoga practice in substance. Merely broader volume is included into the sphere of your feeling and thinking under the character of your 'body'. In Yoga practice mastering in asanas requires to remove muscular blocks, pranayama helps to align energy flows in subtle body, and meditation teaches to concentrate con-sciousness independently from any body, which should not to stop penetration anymore. In Feng Shui practice you have to study the same: how to move furniture or to put fans in proper places that general structure of your home allows to relax and spreads your consciousness without impinging sharp corners, emanative 'envenomed shafts'.

Despite popularity of Feng Shui, since Hatha Yoga be-longs to Indian tradition, here we'll describe some basic princi-ples of Vastu that is Indian art of living space construction. Feng Shui makes special reference to correcting means, enabling to improve inferior dwelling, but Vastu is predominantly dedicated to underlying planning. Unfortunately, it's difficult to use Vastu in Western cities, where most people may not plan their flats themselves, though they are free to construct villas. Nevertheless we can take advantage of this knowledge for diagnostic of present accommodation and relative correction of our own proper habits that to live and practice there specifically better. At least we can choose the direction of that wall, which we are going to use for asana mastering.

Certainly Vastu of Yoga Shala (or just Yoga hall) takes into account the directions, limited by walls, and your choice of Yoga-room depends on general configuration of building. The walls are considered to be auspicious, if they are faced East or North, particular the north-east corner. Namely this direction is the best as a special place, which is intended to lead for Yoga practice and meditation. In India the Puja room (where they perform rituals) is located in the center of house, but north-east corner is also possible for divine worship, however it is not appropriated in other directions. Properly, if you are serious in Yoga and devote your progress to Lord in any favorite form then practice will be important part of daily Puja.

It is essential also to puzzle out the common features of Vastu Purusha Mandala as a concept, which based on feeling of vibrating inner space in the house. Ancient Hindu not so much believed, how much experienced, that each place on the ground surface possesses peculiar vibration, therefore they selected the site for construction very carefully. Every place has some quality of life and represents some energetic entity, which were called as the Purusha (Person) by Hindus. He was regarded with reverence as the certain deity of house, and Hindus held exclusive ceremony, approached him with prayer and asked him to turn according to the proper direction. After this rite Vastu Purusha (Spirit of House) proved to keep his head on north-east corner and his feet in the opposite south-west corner. It is not difficult to relate that Puja room was located directly in the Purusha's heart or head.

It is really interesting for us that the vertical axis of Purusha's body is found in horizontal and his Sushumna is oriented from one corner to another one. Thus, Chakras in Purusha's subtle body situated on diagonal of house, and they work as centers of energy's conversion. Eventually it is obtained that the highest (cranial) Purusha's Chakras, which produces the most subtle and extreme vibrations are also located in north-east corner. For instance, master of Vastu, Suresh Pavar from Mysore, recommended even to add on building to north-east direction. As a result, if you constructed the energy structure of your house correctly, then it's highest point will be found north-eastwardly. Surely, mastering asanas with support of walls in north-east corner, you'll get maximal effect from Yoga practice.

In greater detail the principles of Vastu were described in my other book *"Vastu – Indian Feng Shui. Garlands from Mythic Flowerage"*, published in Russian (Saint-Petersburg, 2004). There I gave special attention to cultivation of Indian plants in Western doors. Certainly, some citizens took advantage of that book and made small jangles or garden in window aperture of Puja room, and these plantings improved tone for Yoga occupation. Generally alfresco the choice of energy field is also determined by vertical energy flow, directed by trees or rocks. However we will come back to this topic, when we pass from practice with support of wall on improvisation with support of an uneven surface of rocks. That has relation to development area in practice, while we are going to sort out its background.

'Support' – Invitation to Development

Not only exchanging the area of support in asanas from feet to palms radically shifts the level of practice on the whole, but also exchanging the surface of support itself shifts the quality of practical consciousness. Most Hatha Yoga instructors, especially among Iyengar-style practitioners, use wall for the mastery of asanas on different levels both the simplest and complicated one. The wall works as support in both cases: at asanas' simplification in Yoga-therapy or at advanced practice in researching for additional variations. However there is the principal difference between interaction with the wall and employment of other subsidiary means (ropes, blocks, rollers etc.). The fact is that dependence doesn't arise but challenge guides the way for the further development. Nevertheless it should be mentioned, which other props could be entered into practice as well as the reason why it would be better to restrict oneself to the wall only instead of anything else.

In the first instance let us settle upon the basic idea for using all props and take a good look at real case in the practice

24

by B.K.S. Iyengar himself. Once an aged philosopher was leaded to Yoga Shala since he became so weak that already could not move without exterior help by his disciples. Yoga teacher examined a patient, then prescribed him hardest standing asanas, and explained: 'He will perform them supine!' In other words practice started from a simple imagination of mastering these postures by himself, then an imitation of external forms were added to their projection, while finally the oldster was able to perfect asanas really standing. This day a stretch of three months he left Iyengar's Yoga Shala, walking on his own foot by his lonesome. It is quite easy to answer the question how was such a miracle possible, just enough to refresh memory about interconnection between body, energy and consciousness.

In a broad manner all that is well-known not only in the ancient Yoga but also in the modern psychology. When we represent ourselves in a specific pose, then the imaginative power displaces energy body similar to actual form, because subtle body falls for mental influence easier than physical body. But because namely energy flows govern all physiological functions, body is going through changing, which is necessary for real execute of the posture. Otherwise, the first idea takes shape in an image then the image incarnates into the thing. In such a way indeed it is possible to prepare for asana practice even in the invalid's wheel chair, say nothing of less tough lucks. Likewise you can force yourself to get over inertial resistance rather simple laziness, since as you know the most difficult in Yoga is to spread mat and enter upon practice. At the beginning try to spread mat and to lay down that "indulge in reverie" on Yoga practice. Surely sooner or later the imagination will start to externalize oneself into life, since body will intend to move completely naturally...

Let us return to props or subsidiary means. One may ask how they could be entered into practice at all, because somebody will hardly believe that in the ancient times Yoga was mastered with the help of chairs. The case is the personal fate of Iyengar himself as well as his guru Krishnamacharya's interest in development in the area of Yoga-therapy. Namely Krishnamacharya input in use subsidiary means for alleviation learning advanced asanas at the very beginning, and this tendency became the characteristic feature of Iyengar Yoga. Deficiency of sitting meditations in Iyengar's system is also raised to Krishnamacharya's idea that asana practice as such lets to improve the self-consciousness power. But the only person who had firsthand knowledge of unreal attempts to take Yoga by "assault" he could enter so many auxiliaries into usual Yoga practice and make special reference to "art of prudence", up to and including idea of asana imitation by feeble. Owing to Iyengar's admission, he learned the most advanced poses not in the course of regular and long-term engagement but just before demonstrations. In any such situation it was important to perform asana faultlessly at the very first attempt though explanation was reduced to two-three brief denotations.

At the first meeting Krishnamacharya shown Iyengar just some simple asanas, but he was so weak after many diseases in the childhood, that soon teacher lost any interest to him. Yet it fortuned that few days before International Yoga Conference the best disciple escaped Krishnamacharya's Yoga Shala. Nobody was ready to demonstrate yogic postures and guru gave attention to Iyengar again. Next morning he showed him about thirty-forty basic asanas at the same time, one after another, and said shortly: 'You must do it'. There was no any other option in this situation. Iyengar got few days only to master asanas till the very perfection and demonstrate on the conference. During the show he fell all over himself so tears appeared from the eyes. Demonstration passed and knocked its opponent for a loop, and teacher confided that he didn't expect such a result. That event connected Iyengar's life with Yoga forever; however he paid the extreme price and suffered from pain in the whole body for long months.

That is why Iyengar tried to discover new methods when he started to teach Yoga himself that traumatize his disciples on no account. Therefore not only in classes on Yoga-therapy but also commonly he prescribed for beginners a lot of props. Of course, the props establish subsidiary points of support for body; they make asana accomplishment easier and help to correct it more properly. But all that aids and appliances became habitual in such a degree, that anybody may call them the feature of Iyengar-style. Even if you perform the advanced asana like Pincha Mayurasana (forearm balance) perfectly, you should learn the special technique how to master the same posture with the help of block hold between palms, etc. It seems the same regarding to the wall: technical development of asanas at the wall made a peculiar kind of art. Then wall is not a support anymore but means of evolution by practice. And yet there is one amount of invention.

For the matter of meditative component of asana practice, this was noticed above. As you know the main goal of meditation is *citta vritti nirodha* that is 'elimination of whirls inside of consciousness'. Put the other way round, consciousness is purified step by step from any conceptions, fades into blank self-actualization. When meditation becomes a part of asana practice, then it is required to keep some posture. You should completely relax your whole body and narrow down its perception to the single grasp of this unique form. In the process you can take into consideration some details of alignment bodily position but then they should be dissolved in consciousness. However introduction of all possible ropes, blocks, chairs, blankets and other inconceivable compositions into bodily form never will give you to do the last step… But the wall is the clean surface!

Part II.
Practice: Montage of Asanas

Outsets we shall distinguish asanas discretely, that quite satisfy the requirements of Iyengar' style. In static practice one should take into consideration cross impact of asanas at their combined influences on the body, and still they are spaced from each other. Asana is microcosm, where you should establish an order without spot or wrinkle, adjusting position and condition of every part and even a cell of your body. This is a reason that asanas' arrangement is secondary, and when you are coming to Yoga-hall it is difficult to dope out, if instructor suggests to perform in the beginning simple forward bend or hand-stand. Virtually inimitable pattern of asanas is taken shape at every lesson, though they emphasize one another in some measure. Eventually asanas' classification which is suggested here is derived; and you may grade the sequence in other easy-to-handle way.

Notwithstanding you should take into account some rules of asanas' combinations. If you have ahead nobody except unanswered wall, then the simplest method 'not to harm' is the following. Perform any posture for alignment and relaxation after every asana. It is necessary to keep neutral position unless and

until you feel that all tracery consisting from many stress re-
gions, appeared at the mastering the previous asana, have already vanished into thin air. Then you can proceed to forming-
up forthcoming asana. Even if you construct completely wrong
sequence, effects from 'misalignment' will not accumulate, and
you will escape trauma, which would be inevitable otherwise. All
that is working for some period, which is enough to learn how to
organize correct self-practice. Don't hope for omnipotence of
relaxation; don't ride Yoga on assumption of momentary mood.

The best pose to be appropriated for relaxation after a
particular asana depends on body position. If you are standing,
you can come back to Tadasana and aline the body. Otherwise
you can perform Utkatasana that is forward bend with elbow
lock. If you are sitting, it would be better to relax in Darnikasana
or 'child pose': sitting on your knees you should bend forward,
put stomach on thigh and forehead on floor, and place hands
along legs. Certainly here you can use for alignment any symmetrical meditative asana like Padmasana, Vajrasana or their
simplified versions. If you are lying on the back, then you can
naturally perform Shavasana or 'corpse pose': spine and head
are in-line; straight arms and legs are diverted from body at an
acute angle. If you are lying on the abdomen, it is not necessary
to turn. You can relax in Makarasana like 'crocodile': put your
forehead down on hands crossed before head and separate extended legs aside, setting footsteps' interior edges on the floor.

Few among us have plenty of time that they take the liberty to spend so long breaks even during practice. Indeed in such a situation at the start your exercises will be limited by several asanas in total. Surely this approach has undeniable advantage for realization of going processes outside, but incidence will be hardly remarkable inside of the body at all. For a lot of pragmatic people, although they need relaxation in the first instance, the abovementioned sounds as something unsuitable. How to act when you wish to maintain the dynamical style of practice? There is some other way, which renders assistance to fulfill asana by asana; and that is the 'contra-posture' principle. You need to adopt the certain skills and analytical powers, but usually it is simply to observe the method. Merely you keep a check on compensation influences: for example, bend is next to arch, etc. But at the present let us examine asanas themselves.

Types of Body Pressure onto Wall

Since the 'wall' is not just a wall for us but the 'prop' leading to transcendence, therefore further we are going to envisage Hatha Yoga as psychic technique. That is not the case that you merely adjust the body, why it would look superior and function smooth-running. No doubt it is essential too but still absolutely insufficient. It is more important that you learn how to take advantage of methods which hopes to influence body for the purpose of transformation through entire personality, including feeling, thinking and spirituality. So, you must aspire not to master advanced asanas faster, but to fulfill simplest asanas with perfect self-awareness. No need to perform handstand 'askance', even though body seems 'dead straight' from external view. The question is what you are feeling at the moment, whatever your mind is concerned with, what extent your consciousness is merged into divine. So, along the strike of exposition on technical details we shall note their action on systemic condition.

According to words by one instructor of Hatha Yoga every possible asanas' classification is the effort 'to press multifaceted entity inside square box'. Needless to say, it is not necessary to squeeze it there. Simply and solely keep in your mind that any common description possesses a high potential; and optionally you can evolve it under the very different reflex angles, no matter how extensively and no matter how extensively and sweepingly. Such a schema should be accepted as a working model, which is able to fulfill required operation in fixed stage, while you replace it by something more appropriate. Don't become attached to exterior forms, whether it is mental definition or physical ability to do anything perfectly. Today you perform a technique delightfully, but in the case if you are developing tomorrow you can discover that it is not requisite without theatrics and even interfering. It is equally true for typology: in advance keep more emptiness or free space. You will need it for progression and accumulating of your own experience.

As for the principle of given classification, we are going to discriminate asana's types owing to distinctive bodily pressure onto vertical surface at poses' performance against the wall. Although the wall is the very simplest thing, it proves that interaction between you and wall passing rich in point of fact. Sometimes its evenness is the most important, but sometimes its stability is more important and so on. You need to spread body on the wall's surface for mastering some asanas, but you need to skim the same wall by fingertips only for mastering other asanas. Moreover you will be interested in wall's extension till one or another level; in this case solid surface is not necessary, just distinctive object is required in the space above horizontal plane. The wall is always good enough for this purpose because it serves as such an object at any level. Well, let us see what we are able to do specifically relying on these general principles.

Axial Alignment inside of Body

As you know 'monkey' became 'human being' when one upraised from all fours, straightened back, reared head and looked around, keeping balance on total of two feet. And now to be serious hitherto perfection of vertical position leaves much to be desired. Modern man suffers from chronic stoop, blocking connection between lower and higher centers. As a result pristine instincts live owing to their own nature, determining body to commit spontaneous deeds; visionary schemes hulk up vainly at head; and non-processed splendid feeling glimmers in cramped chest. There's no doubt about prolongation of vertical axis beyond body up and down. As a matter of fact even that part of personality, which confined from top to heels, doesn't manage according to conception of straight line. But axis refers to elemental geometric constructions both ideally and in flesh.

Habit to make sideways of corpus is destructive also. When you put all the weight of body on one leg then this side is cramped while opposite side is bagged out of control. At this rate the balance between Ida and Pingala is broken, that's why you lose sense of proportion externals of activity and passivity, say nothing of extrusion of inner organs. Of course, we should move and currently assume asymmetrical positions. That means liberty of action includes namely possibility to deviate from neutral position and come back to axis again to perform new actions. Otherwise all structure would be permanently deformed. So, when we start Yoga practice, the wall helps us for alignment of vertical body position as such. We seek for performing of Tadasana and setting of right angles at forward bending.

Tadasana – 'Rock' Posture

When you are standing straight and stable like an inviolable rock, then your body becomes light and clarity appears in your consciousness. It is important to align the body in vertical from all directions, reclining against the wall alternatively back, side and forehead. It stands to reason that every time you should recede from the wall one step back and try to feel and keep the vertical without any support. Resting against the wall there is no need to approach a complete contact between your back and the wall, since a spine is certainly slightly curved. But measure and course of its incurvation are under the question; and here the wall helps to do the next three correct movements that to put back into alignment.

Outthrust of tail bone forward-up lets you to spread lumbar on the wall, eliminates cramp, which sooner or later inevitably results in rheumatism and backache. Legs ought to get over that position, because it requires little bit other opening of hips than habitual. Brace yourselves by arm crosswise behind shoulders and expand back; whereupon force shoulders apart aside and slightly down, opening chest. It is important to turn shoulders not backwards, as usually anybody undertakes to perform, constricting spinal column and creating tension in chest. You should move shoulders namely every which way; also your back and chest are found stretched and relaxed equally. Finally don't try to press your neck against the wall, overturning your head upwards. But on the contrary make an effort to achieve that result by extension of neck upwards, as if you would be pulled from crown of head. In the process chin will come down slightly; and this motion will cause relaxation of your throat.

After experiencing every inch of spinal column from the top to the bottom you should recoil one step from the wall and try to maintain the vertical position succeeded by means of wall now with a help of muscles only. Then come back to wall again and check your sensations. Surely, you don't need to walk as a stick returning to your daily life likewise you pass on execution of other asanas continuing practice. Nevertheless Tadasana is the basic pose for standing relaxation; and it serves as the primary position throughout standing asanas. Good idea to repeat Tadasana after performing any other pose that test an alignment of body, whereupon you may proceed to sequent asana.

Regular control of vertical is also beneficial in the real life because it improves your current conditions such as self-confidence, equability during manifestation of feelings, stability of subjective attitude in business stream. From psychological point of view Tadasana promotes to form certain inner 'column', that is the base of a character, but on the energy level it constructs the central axis. Entire energy structure consisting from subtle bodies, channels and centers is orientated in correspondence to the axis. The appropriation of axis must become the first object of your attention. Hereafter you will gradually accustom to operate with feeling of axis in the worldly life, arranging with relation to vertical all things and connections around.

There are some details in forming of Tadasana which are imperceptible outwardly to anybody untutored in Yoga, but visible to somebody who knows on his own experience how an internal work reflects into an exterior shape. At the perfect weight distribution on footsteps the pressure is fallen not within toes or heels, but directly on the middle point which is well-known in acupuncture. In order to find the place you should make an effort to keep footsteps in contact with floor area: arise your toes, set them apart, and then put them down in a spread state. At these movements skin on backside of footstep is shifted outwards. Besides you can do the series of turning by palms outward and return that set up thoracic girdle strictly over hips. It is important to perform this motion either side that to catch perfect mid position. Likewise temporary body bending with slow return to Tadasana can help to feel vertical.

A criterion for the correct fulfillment of the pose is perfect balance, when gravitational center is not dislocated. Similar to skyscraper, your corpus neither falls nor even quakes. It is essential to get irreproachable vertical position going to realize inverted asana later. Body should get the same position in Shirshasana (headstand) as in Tadasana, especially the form of legs and feet. If you are able to stand straightly on your feet, then it will not be difficult for you to stand straightly on your top anymore. Alternatively the mastering of headstand has unconditional value for getting into the habit the standing straight on your feet. You see, performing headstand you begin to observe such details which went into the sub-consciousness long ago during millennial feet-stand practice. Psychoanalysts confirm that everything is mixed in this sphere and nothing can be preserve directly as it was. As a result the skill of straight walking is liable to all kinds of extraneous influences and incrustations.

Sidelong Alignment

As it was mentioned above you can prepare yourselves for the aligning body in Tadasana also with reclining against the wall by each side or with resting upon the wall by forehead. In both cases the vertical is saved, though it is felt inside of body and working in another way. The sidelong alignment helps to accent the function of lateral canals Ida and Pingala, which are parallel with central axis.

Try to stand against the wall sideward pressing exterior edge of footstep close to the wall as far as possible (Photo 1). You will be required to take stronger purchase on the opposite leg, since a thrust of the hip against the walls will push your corpus outward. Simultaneously arise up the arm nearest to the wall, turning palm and pressing it onto the surface, and merely stretch down another arm, pulling it along the corpus. Thus the whole lateral line of your body is extended along the wall from foot to palm. In this position the exposed side of the body is extremely stretched and compressed; on the contrary, the interior side is completely relaxed and expanded, spreading-eagle on the wall. The alternation of left and right sides renders a possibility to work at energy streams going through both lateral canals namely Ida and Pingala. Say nothing of the influence on tissues and organs by successive exertion and relaxation.

The question is what really depends on these uncomplicated actions in your practice as well what is obviously changing in your daily life. Even if you will merely try to stand against the wall by one and another side, then you will feel the remarkable difference between both sides of your body. This is the case; they are opposite and mutually complementary. It is well-known from different functions of left and right brains likewise from operation of solar and lunar channels in the slender body. Theoretically both sides must be compensated, and on physical layer it reflects in symmetrical movements. However in the vast majority people possess one-sided view on current circumstances and usually they reproduce one-dimensional behavior. All asymmetrical asanas are always mastered on both sides that you would achieve alignment starting from this simplest stand.

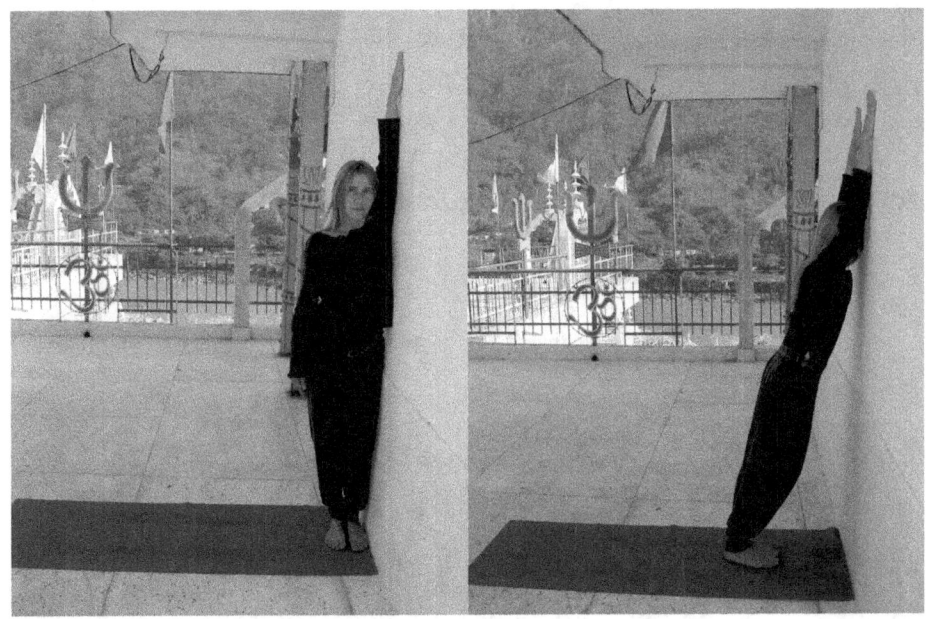

Photos 1-2

There are some details in working out the literal aligning also such as transferring of pressure onto the outer side of footstep and tightening of the inner side. Be sure, the case in hand is mental effort which produces a whisk of tissues in flesh. Don't try to perform this exercise moving legs up and down. Moreover you should strive to work by both legs in each position, but not only with the help of outer leg. Being retained against wall by one and another side, you will work out both footsteps in different ways. But totally the entire body becomes stressed from outside and relaxed inside. Thus the body attains exact borders, and all necessary processes happen at the limits naturally.

You can add this posture into many asanas' complexes which are suitable for elimination of all superfluous arches, for example arches in feet and back (Tadasana) or arches in palms at the pressure by hands against the wall (vertical variation of Dandasana). But it is worthy of special mention underneath.

Frontal Extension of Body

Now you vertical structure has already become similar to real column which is more stable then original axis. However you should also feel the frontal line of the body for better forming of inner volume. You see, in the common standing position and especially when back is close to the wall almost the whole weight of the body suppresses the spine that is back side only. Even if you perform lateral alignment then you give attention to Ida and Pingala in the spine column, therefore your concentration moves to your back naturally. It is happening also in the case if you sink on your heels, but such a sinking is fatal at spontaneous efforts to maintain posture without special correction of feet. This situation is quite natural therefore you have to assume the next specific position for working out the front line.

Stand opposite the wall, recoil one step backward, maintain straight corpus from heels to top, and lean forehead unto the wall. Don't touch the wall by any other point of your body as well don't push the wall by the forehead since this position is irrelevant to category of 'thrusts'. The distance between your feet and the wall should be enough that you could feel a tension in the front line of the body. But there should not be too much free space otherwise you'll incline to fall limb and bone on the wall. So, you are standing on own legs firmly, moreover you are pushing the floor by your feet that preferably extract all forward side of your body. On this evidence your arms could assume either position: pull them upwards pressing palms against the wall (Photo 2) or make elbow lock setting palms on elbows crosswise (Photo 3). These variations are different according to their ability for combination with other postures in sequences.

Outstretching arms you distantly commence to prepare your body for handstand producing a pressure on palms and extending body in line. For this reason it is advantageous to interchange that position and Utkatasana or forward bending with putting palms before feet (when flexibility allows it). Beyond all doubt afterwards you will press into handstand namely from this pose. As an intermediate link in the exercises for mastering shoulder's position you can use also Adho Mukha Shvanasana or 'down facing dog' in common yogic parlance. In this posture palms and feet thrust against the floor so far that tail bone forms the corner of a triangle. It is no wonder that later we will come back to this standard asana very often. But the most natural movement to the next pose is the passage to arms' position with a thrust into the floor by elbows.

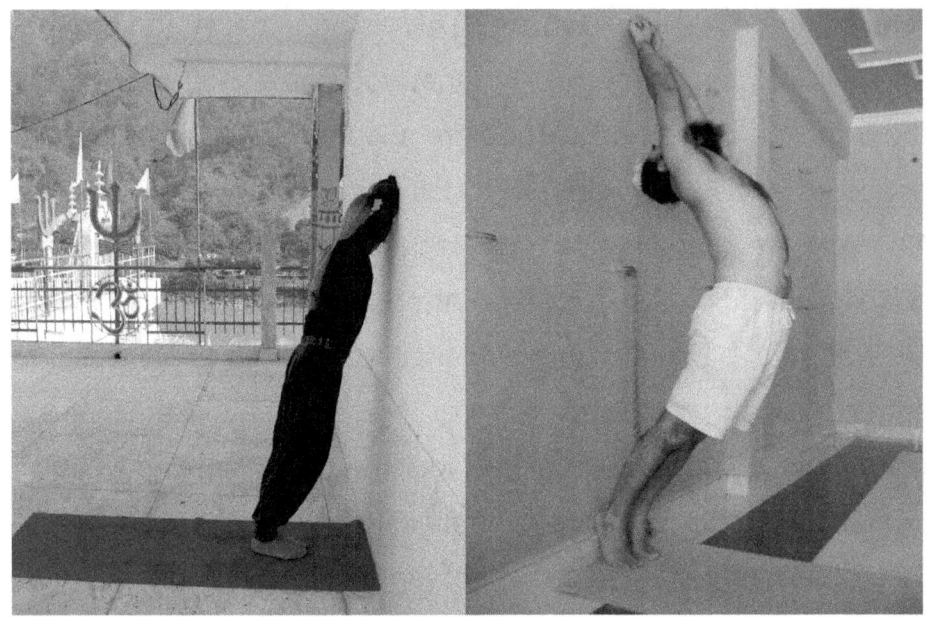

Photos 3-4

An alternative pose with elbow lock is well suited to the relaxation after Tadasana, especially if you deepened the extension of your back with arching. For instance, if you hold a hook overhead and arch all your body pushing off the wall by heels as strong as possible standing with your back to the wall (Photo 4). Then turn heading forward to the wall and put forehead and elbows on its surface. Then slightly bend your knees and completely relax you chest, but after that again straighten and stretch your legs. This method operates in many asanas with wall; hence it is desirable to master it well in primary version. If you are not able to stretch your body correctly, then it's always better to wait before performing the ideal posture and to relax in approximate pose. Finally it makes sense to go through every movement in reverse order: put both hands upwards, return to Tadasana with your back to wall, and recoil from wall. Repetition from the end to the beginning is among basic methods which are suitable for mastery of adjoining positions too.

Let us add to the pattern asanas apart from the wall. You will remember that thrust by palms combined with Utkatasana (foreword bending) and Adho Mukha Shvanasana (down facing dog) with straight arms. It is preferable to repeat both asanas with elbow lock. Doing forward bend you should extend straightback but turn off shoulders down to loins to replace them upwards. It is essential to control this movement, since everybody has tendency to squeeze neck by shoulders in the position, but that is wrong. 'Down facing dog' is mastering in the same way, though you push the floor by elbows instead palms. Setting up and withholding of such a triangle is much harder work.

Hands at Right Angle

At present you may set about alignment of your body not against the wall but in parallel with the wall, and by this time that demands more advanced vertical feeling. It will be observed, that these postures seem illusory simple. However even Indian Yoga-teacher boggled his first attempt preparing himself to demonstrate them in front of camera. When we are standing in front of the wall in some distance, there is an alternative approach to shape right angles with the help of limbs. Specifically we can use both arms or legs or one of them, in what connection we can turn back, face or side against the wall. However forward bending with pressing palms or feet on the wall is more like 'thrust against the wall', and preferably we'll give consideration to this type of poses underneath. It is clear, that each several poses lead the way for the whole chain of asanas, similar in appearance and attractive for construction of new sequences.

Stand in front of the wall at arms length and put your palms on the wall on the level of your shoulders (Photo 5). But don't just stand, because you should produce a pressure to the wall by hands, which provokes in return even stretch in all your body that promotes a formal alignment. This position is nothing else than turned around 90 degrees Dandasana, or the thrust against the floor by straight arms with holding of your body in one line. It makes sense to alternate this thrust against wall and the classical 'stick' pose. You can improve standard Dandasana with support of the wall too, merely putting feet on the wall at your shoulders' level. Then inversely you are pushing floor by straight arms and all your body is orientated true-horizontal. Interchange of these positions lets us achieve a clear feeling, which muscles are working for maintaining each position.

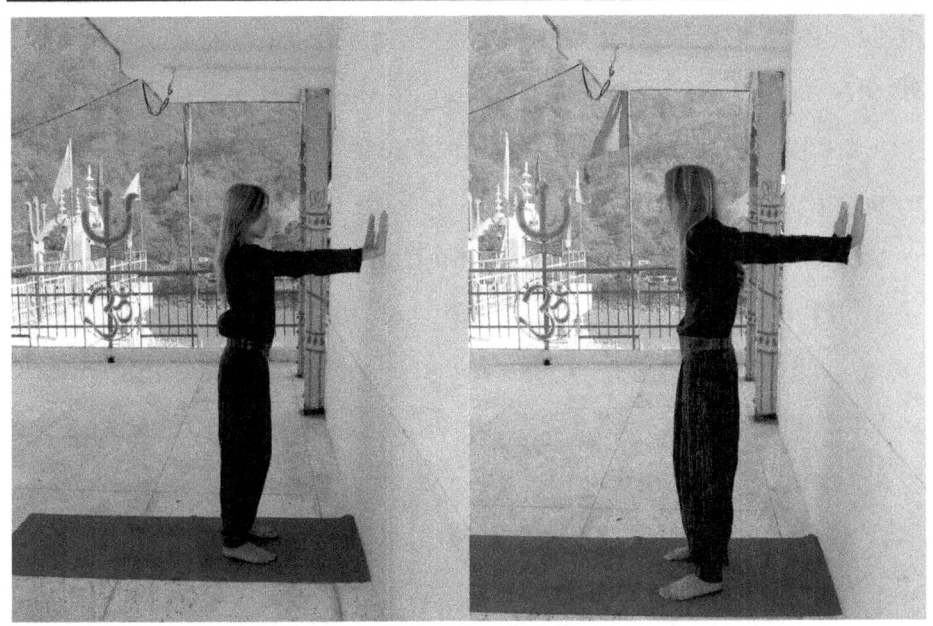

Photos 5-6

Hereafter turn with your back to the wall and assume the mirror position in reference to the previous pose, namely fix your palms on the wall at the level of shoulders (Photo 6). It will be not simple to do it at your leisure, however this posture renders a possibility to develop shoulder joints and open thoracic cage what is beneficial when you will run through more complicated asanas. It's better to start standing sideward against the wall, press palm of one hand to the surface, and lay middle finger true-vertical. Then turn back on the wall and lead another hand to the same position. Probably, in this case you will need extraneous help not only to remove hand back but also to open shoulders under light pressure on them from the front (sometimes it's enough just to touch with fingers). At that process skin will be displaced from your shoulder backwards and down on your back. Certainly you should make an effort to attain the right angle not so much by arms' strength, but by means of shoulder relaxation and thoracic cage opening.

Herein one could be recommended taking advantage of ropes, although on the whole we'll talk about their employment underneath. But you can accomplish quite simple exercises for development of shoulder joints. Fix two ropes (or one rope in the middle with two free ends) to the hook not too high. Stand with your back to the wall, set throwing hands upon free ends and hang on ropes all over. Then start to perform bends back and forth, and in this process your arms will be intensively hinge in shoulders, furthermore stretching under the body weight. However movements should be completely controlled. Never admit any careless handling with your own body!

Another variation is using ropes fixed higher then your head and with exterior assistance. Stand with your back to the wall in some distance, set arising hands upon free ends, and slightly hang on ropes foreword. Assistant must stand behind you, hang on ropes just above your hands, and put arising foot between your shoulder blades. The foot pressure should be intended in a greater measure upwards than forward. Also the pushing should be very careful that stretching would be soft and gradual. An assistant may slightly pull your hands back that you could relax perfectly without any personal efforts to arching.

Legs at Right Angle

Certainly you can not put both legs on the wall at the right angle, provided that you don't sit on the floor. Such a position here you will use in order to admeasure a proper distance from the wall only. It is necessary to stand one leg on the wall correctly; otherwise you will never succeed in the right angle. Besides you can use the preliminary sitting pose to correct and remember the right position of hips. Nevertheless the sitting posture with your face against the wall, straight legs and feet pressing on the wall deserves attention as such also. Namely this pose serves as the original location for many asanas relating to thrusts on the wall. Never fear if you will stay on this point since it will be useful further. But we continue to examine standing asanas and vertical alignment in parallel with surface of wall.

A balancing asana, when you are standing on one leg and arising another leg as high as possible holding big toe by homonymous hand, is called Utthita Hasta Padangushtasana (Photo 7). It is easier to do it standing with your back against the wall especially if you proceed to the next variation and take arising leg aside. However the sense of making this motion with your face against the wall is namely that you master the right angle between your leg and straight your spine with horizontal line of hips. If you are standing with your back against the wall, you don't give attention to these details because they become proper by themselves. But standing with your face against the wall you are required to accomplish the task more consciously.

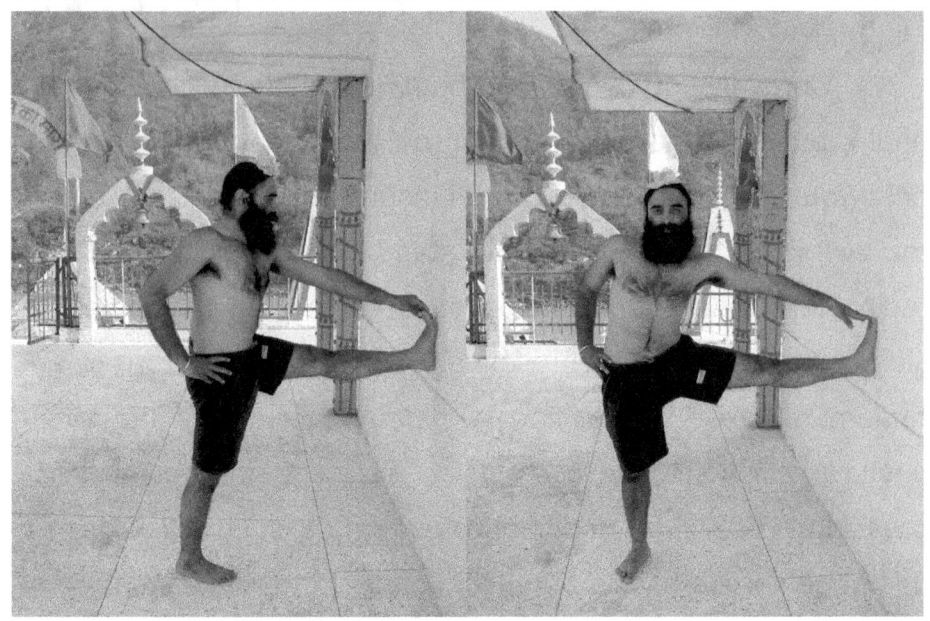

Photos 7-8

In order to admeasure the right distance from the wall exactly you should sit down on the floor and thrust your footsteps against the wall. Then bend your legs and stand up directly at the same place where you were sitting a moment ago. Now you should bend downward, grasp one footstep from outside by palm, straighten trunk arising the bended leg, and erect this leg finally putting your foot on the wall. If your hips are warped then it makes sense to repeat the last movement one more time. Slightly bend your upper leg, correct normal position of hips, and straighten the leg again. But your ability to master the right angle without changing of hand location depends on proportions of your body. In the event that lengths of your arms and legs disproportionate, you have to correct the point of hold-fast. Be careful that return your foot on the floor with the help of your hand also or do it very slowly and consciously, don't throw your leg down out of control.

The following asana is performing in much the same way but in this case you are standing with your side against the wall (Photo 8). This pose can be very difficult for beginners whose hips are not opened that means their hip joints are not developed. Don't force events because you can use for opening of hips other asanas with better effect. At the moment just form an estimate of your posture and feel measure of defect. At this rate it is more easily to work out the asana with your back to the wall. Especially if Yoga-teacher can assistant you, pushing one of your shoulders to the wall and turning your opposite leg aside and upward. The right angle is important for your body alignment but really the higher is your leg the more advanced is asana. In the process your leg and corpus should be in the plane with the wall, while the arising of leg in front of the face is a completely different asana.

At the limit carrying the last asana to extreme, you achieve both forward and cross splits in vertical plane, balancing on one leg. At the beginning you should keep these forms flat and plain in your imagination at least under the character of reference. But when the angle between your legs will become obtuse, then you will get an auxiliary facility to use the wall rather the column. So, turn your face to the column, press both opened legs as close as possible to the surface, and pull your body to upper leg, arming the column. It is far from something out-of-limit, and I observed in Mysore Yoga Mandala how many western students were doing this (Photo 8-a).

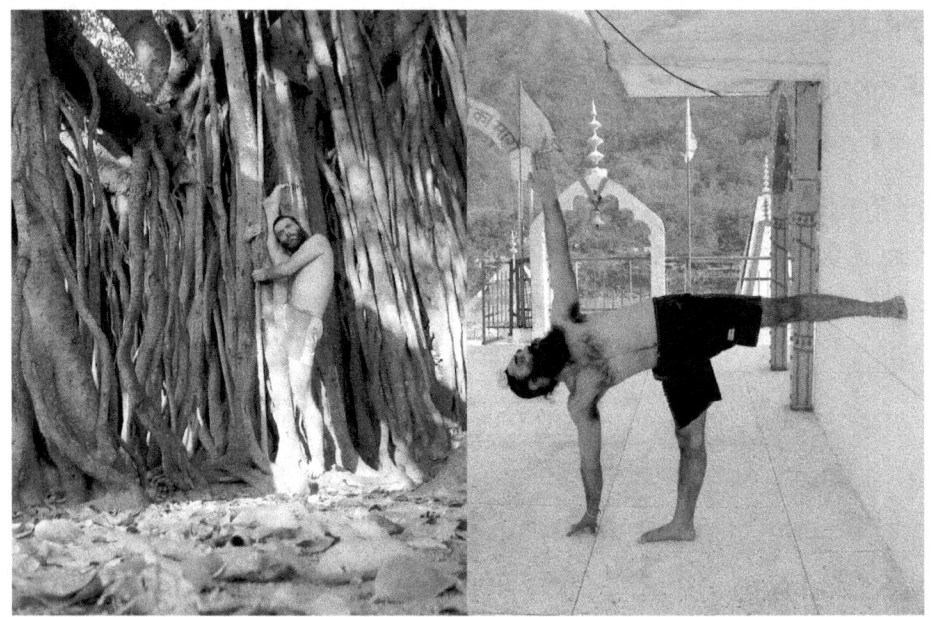

Photos 8(a)–9

Attempt 'to Stand on the Wall' with One Leg

Finally it sticks out a mile that in the last variation the body position is similar to Ardha Chandrasana, or 'half-moon' (Photo 9). We can master this pose with support of the wall also, just making quarter turn in space. Now a stationary foot is standing on the wall, entire body is parallel to the floor, and foot and hand (which pressed the wall in previous pose) are stand-ing on the floor. At the same time an opposite arm is arising upwards, that as a result both arms form straight line and face is turned up to ceiling. You can alternate both described postures on both sides, eliciting the effect of indifference to horizontal and vertical. See, your body keeps the same form but preserves it by different means. Needless to say in this connection right angles are performing catholically and much deeper, so the effect becomes evident much faster.

It will be observed that you can develop horizontal position with your back or abdomen against the wall too. In the first instance your body is more opened for exterior assistance, but in the latter case you get more options for correction by your own forces. But we will come back later to this asana adding variation with spine twisting at the body turning to opposite side. This pose belongs to complicated thrusts on the wall, and we proceed to this category of asanas just now.

Try-out of Limit Stop and Pressure

At psychological level the case in hand is some self-assertiveness. In balanced state it passes into such excellent capacity as insistence in achievement of positive selected goal. Work with the wall will let you to develop the power of conation or ability to pull strings, if you are too infirm. Conversely the same wall will teach you to reckon with barriers and oppositions, if you are prone to bear heavily on amenable environment improvidently and recklessly. Additionally the wall will instruct you how to search out truthful directions for force exertion that neither fall down in a vacuum mechanically nor undertake to unseat monolithic mountains. In short, at this point the wall answers for working-out a sense of proportion in action on the outside world. In what connection at symbolical level you provide various forms of pressure in terms of changing body position in asanas. As a matter of fact it is possible to press outwards not only with different powers, but in different ways also.

Forward Bending at the Right Angle

Body bending (hips flexion only) with putting limbs on the wall belongs to the category of 'thrust on the wall'. Herein also we have two postures wherein body maintains identical positions though they are differentiated in space orientation simply and solely. Either you stand on your legs while your corpus and arms are stretched in line and expanded (Photo 10), or you stand on your hands and then you get more options for work with legs and hips using an abdominal press (Photo 11). Of course, degrees of pressure on the wall are incommensurable in both cases. In the first instance you are pushing softly to extend your back, but in the latter case the thrust must be extremely rigid otherwise you will not hold the right angle at all.

Nevertheless you shouldn't fear handstand in this position since really it relates to elemental postures. It is enough to abut hands on the floor and to shift from one foot to another walking upwards on the wall, until your legs will make the right angle with the surface of the wall, although at the start the angle maybe more or less oblique. Also it is important to stretch your spine up and to pull your head down and to the wall in order to release cramp between shoulder blades. Never bear heavily on hands in handstand, but to the contrary you ought to push your body upwards. In the current and the previous positions arms don't rest on the floor but work constantly. As it happened at body alignment, herein you see exactly similar forms of asanas, which distinguish in nothing else than space orientation. You can alternate both positions mastering the same form as before.

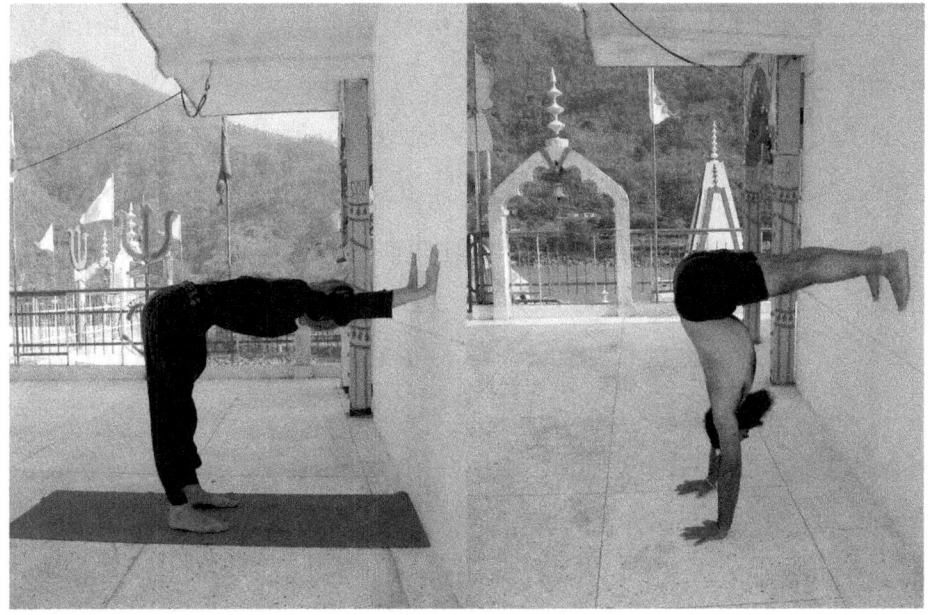

Photos 10-11

Starting from the simple thrust with hands on the wall, again we can refresh memory about such an intermediate position as 'down facing dog'. A cause for its engaging is obvious: 'dog posture' serves as training for complete arm balance, while bending with pushing the wall by hands serves as preparing for handstand with pushing the wall by feet. Thus, 'dog' appears the certain interlink in the chain of complicated asanas. In the capacity of training 'dog posture' you should push off the wall by hands to such an extent that completely eliminate arch in your back. Alternatively we can adopt both thrusts in order to improve 'dog' as such, since it represents the most well-balanced thrust by all fours. Look at the both thrusts against the wall. If we'll connect feet and palms by imaginary line, we'll get the same triangle like in the common 'dog' on the floor. In other words, we optimize that asana in both positions as on inclined plane, orientating head up or down. Whereupon any diagonals come into existence under different reflex angles in our personal space of practice apart from vertical and horizontal lines.

In order to feel the body in these postures much better you can make the following motion, which is very useful for ordinary 'dog' too. Bend your legs in the knees; slightly arise your heels (above floor or aside wall); pull your tail bone back; and then perform the exact triangle again. Standing on the floor you can give special attention to your shoulders, if it is possible to find window sill or another shelf in the wall. Squeeze a wooden block between your palms; and also remove your straight fingers aside; then place your elbows on the shelf and perform already accustomed position. The difference is evident: you thrust not palms but elbows on the wall, and you try to expend your spine backward owing to force which you use for squeezing of block. You pass muscular effort from the palm to the tail bone, and the stronger you squeeze block the easier you align spine. Be careful that no arch, let somebody looks at your back.

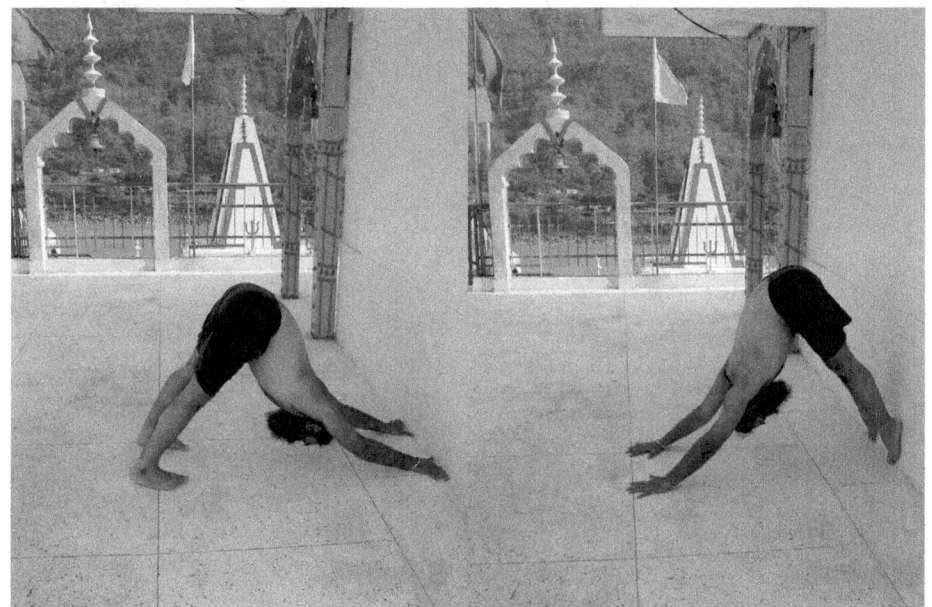

Photos 12-13

Limit Stop at Slipping

Further the wall can serve as the limit stop at performing that asana where hands and feet have tendency to separate sliding over the floor. In the case the wall becomes a limit of horizontal plane while the vertical itself is operative at short interval. There are two failures: both hands and feet move in opposite directions sliding on the floor when you try to keep them at fixed distance; or just feet move from each other when you try to perform some posture 'astride'. But any support of the wall is not too proper to preserve distance between both hands only.

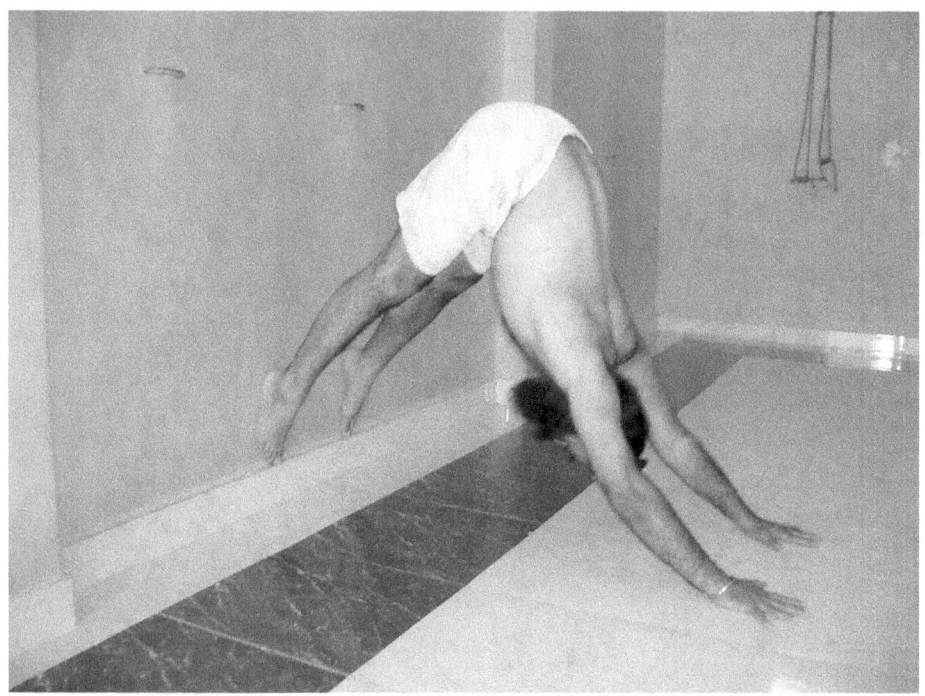

Photo 13(a)

Continually mentioned 'dog' can be mastered on the floor with thrust against the wall by palms or inversely by heels (Photos 12-13). An alternative approach is the thrust by feet at the very low-level above the floor (Photo 13-a); probably you can touch the floor by big toes, if the wall is too slippery. But a criterion of correct performance of asana on rough wall is the measure of legs stretching for the thrust, which doesn't give to slide feet down till floor. You should stand on the wall closely and se-curely, and in that event rather work off an arching back, than maintain straight a spinal column. Your head is pulling to the wall and to the floor simultaneously, while it will touch surface by top of forehead. If you prefer to turn, then push the wall by palms, more properly by hollow between your thumb and finger. Otherwise put the base of your palm on the floor but put the base of your fingers on the edge of cornered block. Keep your palm extended and stretched at the right angle to your arm.

When you master 'triangles' it is convenient to set up the footstep of your back leg against the wall and to line up a whole asana in perpendicular to the wall (Photo 14). 'Triangles' are standard elements of Iyengar-style, and students repeat them by body like physical mantras. The most difficult in performance of correct posture is the opening of your hips that entire body would be really in the plane. Maybe you will need an assistant with rope. The helper should pass the rope between your legs and throw it over both hips against buttocks. Then he pulls one free end backwards, turning the back hip outside, and at the same time he should pull on another free end by another hand, turning the front hip inside. Being alone you can use support of the wall again. At this rate it makes sense to line up 'triangle' with your back close to the wall (Photo 15), being retained against its surface with your small of the back and opening hips by means of exertion and relaxation of required muscles.

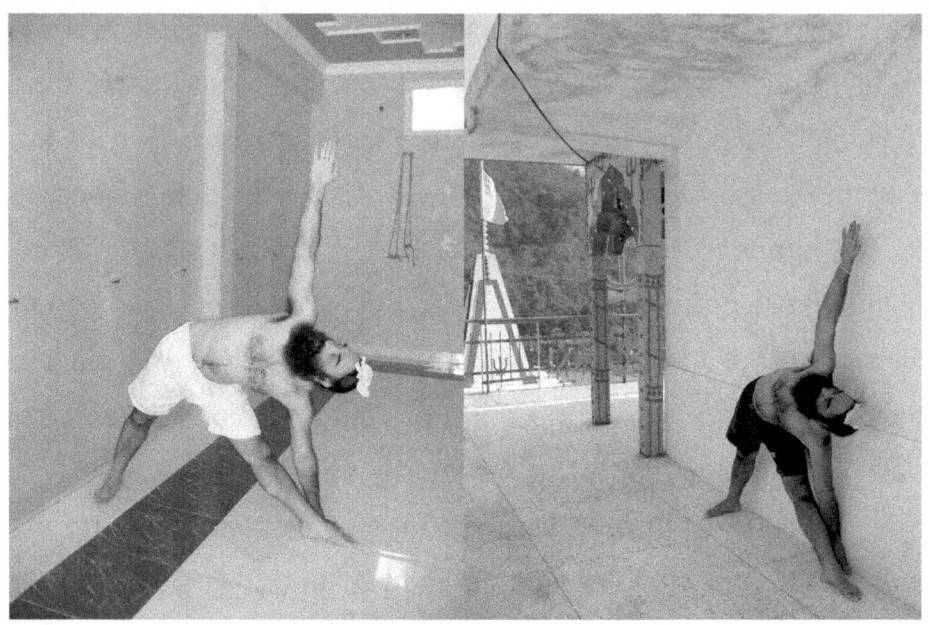

Photos 14-15

Forward Bending with Back Pressure

When you are standing with your back against the wall performing 'triangle' then you can change the side passing through a fulfillment of one more asana that is Prasarita Padottanasana (Photo 16). In that case you need the support of the wall because forward bending forces you to move your hips back but namely this tendency doesn't allow you to bend lower till the very limit. However it is quite difficult to keep balance if you spread your legs aside broadly in vertical plane therefore this asana works as a balancing posture even near the wall. Nevertheless Prasarita Padottanasana helps a lot for opening of your hips if you increase the distance between feet at the same time bending lower with a straight spine. The last-mentioned condition is of critical importance, so you can inure yourself to meet the requirement with help of the next asana. While practicing the pose you need neither hips opening nor balancing that's why you can relax and bring into focus the forward bending.

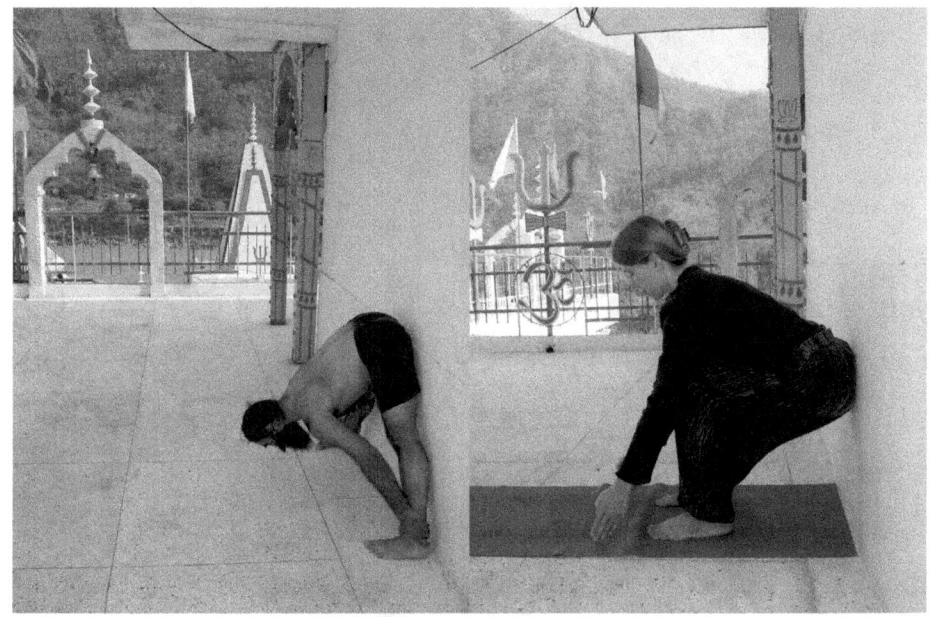

Photos 16-17

In standing position the forward bending is called Padangushtasana if you catch big toes by fingers or Padahastasana if you put palms under footsteps. However the degree of your bending is not important in the preparing variation against the wall. In order to master this posture you should lean your buttocks unto the wall, extend your arms downward and put them on your legs in any distance from the floor. Concentrate on straightening of your back. At the limit you will fold in twain putting your abdomen on your thighs. But don't try to touch knees by forehead otherwise certainly you will round your back. With intent to feel your body in this position firstly you should bend your legs so much that really put your abdomen on the thighs keeping straight spine. Then slowly straighten legs (Photo 17), not bending your back in this procedure but turning your chest upward and still pressing your abdomen against your thighs.

Now you can try to repeat the same movement without support of the wall, then come back to the wall and continue your work with straight legs. However, it's a requested preparation to do simple training motions standing in Tadasana. Separate your heels outwards and try to bend forward working with an external side of feet and without moving your buttocks back. Straightening up you should feel the energy flow springing from footsteps and going through legs to hips. After such a "pumping" of legs channels you should turn with your back against the wall, put your heels within one step from the wall, and abut your tail bone on the wall (Photo 18). As a matter of convenience it is desirable to put a wooden block under the base of toes (Photo 18-a). Then feet and legs will rest at the right angle to each other as in the general standing position. Anyway keep your legs straight, stretch your arms in the direction to feet, bend your body down with a straight spine, and look to your front.

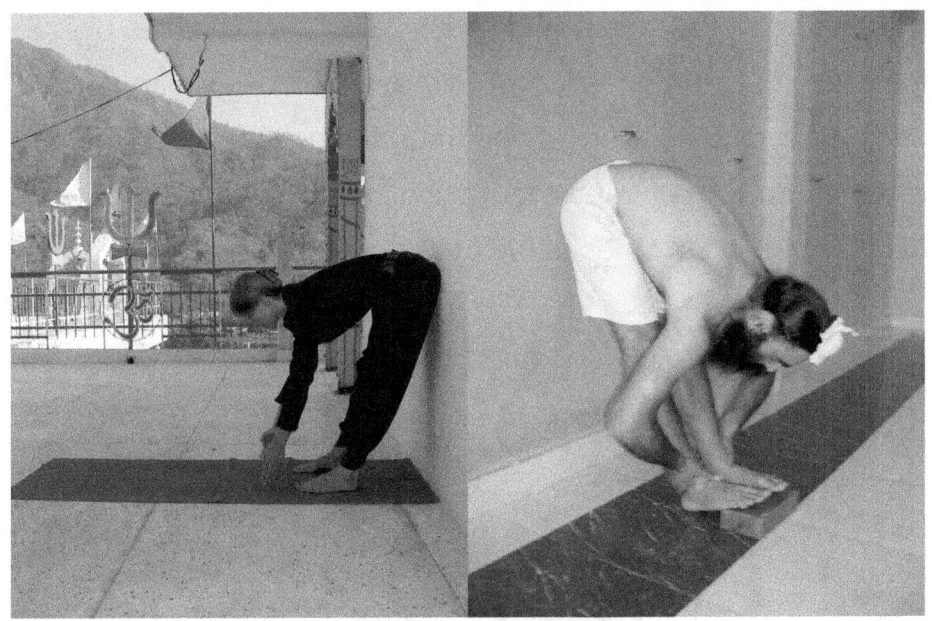

Photos 18-18(a)

In order to deepen the bending you can set your hands on ankles and pull your body to legs (Photo 19). At the same time keep your back straight and try to put an abdomen on thighs, like you carried through formerly with legs bending. After that you should upraise corpus withholding ankles with your hands, and attempt to arch the back. Exactly you don't have to round your back, but in quite opposite way you should arch the spine like for back bending. You can use one more trick which forces your muscles to work. Bend your legs a little bit, hold something like a blanket between an abdomen and thighs, and straighten legs without loosing the blanket. At the process always keep hands on your ankles because you need to master namely this posture. The effort for holding the blanket is directly the effort for the perfection of this asana. However if you feel and understand the work of your muscles quite enough, then it's better to do everything without supplementary props. You see, the less of supports means the better practice.

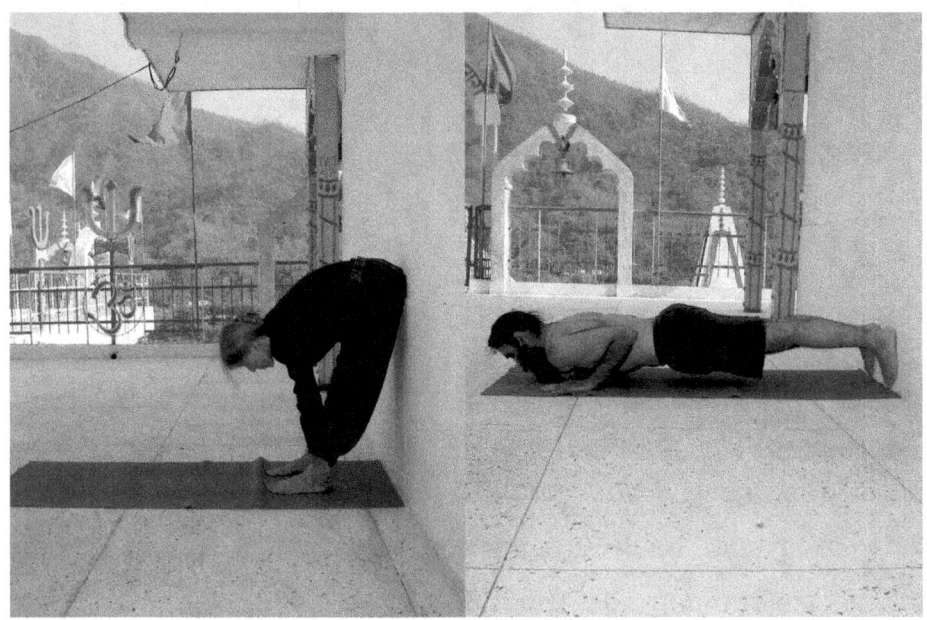

Photos 19-20

Attempts 'to Stand on the Wall' with Both Legs

There are interesting variations mastering the maintaining of the body in horizontal with inversion of space, where the wall serves as a support for feet. Performing Chaturanga Dandasana you should press feet against the wall as if you would 'stand on the wall' in order to stretch an entire body forward (Photo 20). For mastering the advanced asana you should put your feet on the wall at the shoulders' level that all body become in parallel with the floor (Photo 21). The thrust by feet is very useful for the common Dandasana too though not so much, and we have already mentioned this asana above shortly. You see, in this posture feet aren't going to slip and back is straightened easier. On the contrary as we specified above in details firstly you can work out Dandasana standing with your face against the wall, leaning on its surface by palms, and producing at the moment the effort which you need for a thrust on the floor. As a result the wall serves as a support for hands here also.

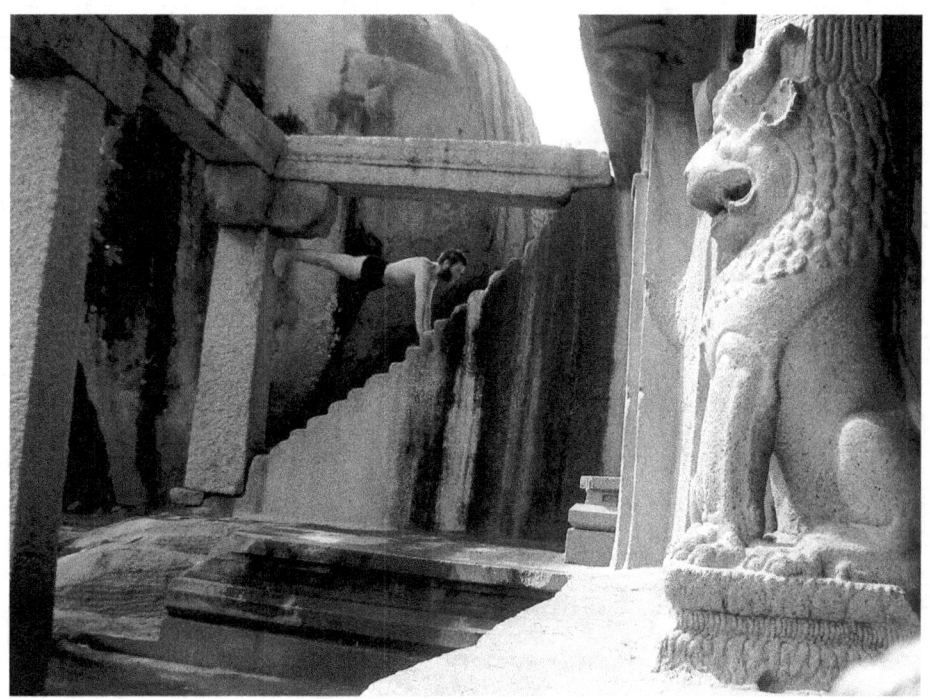

Photo 21

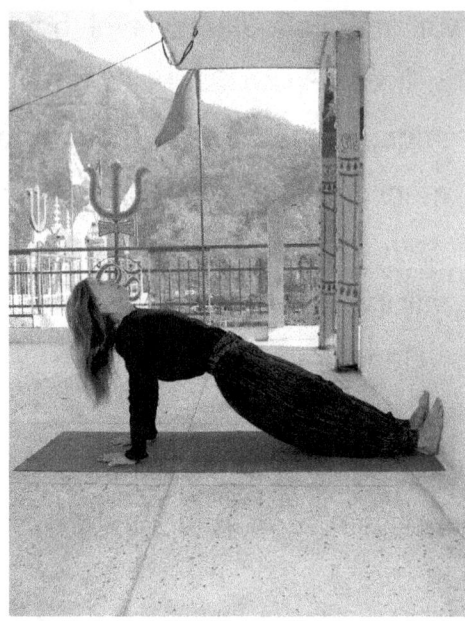

Photo 22

However it is possible to apply the thrust on the wall by feet when you perform asana which is symmetrical to Dandasana. This is the same inclined thrust with straight body but facing up and keeping whole weight on your arms reversed in shoulders. The name of the pose is Purvottanasana (Photo 22). For preparation you should recover sitting on the floor, facing against the wall and pressing it by feet. Remember, how you mastered the pose earlier (before putting one leg on the wall at the right angle). Since there is no need to worry about legs anymore, you can decide two other tasks namely opening of shoulders and inversion of wrists. Going gradually from the simple to the complicated you can do the next sequence of motions. Put your palms behind buttocks turning fingers back and arise hips up till the whole body becomes in one line. Then come down on the floor, make finger lock, reverse the lock and arise straight arms up, as if you push the ceiling with your palms, stretching the body upward. Again come back to the original position, put hands aside buttocks turning fingers forward, and perform Purvottanasana one more time though it will be much harder. Finally put buttocks on the floor and arise straight arms up turning your fingers back as if you would perform handstand on the ceiling.

The last pose requires significant efforts, though extrinsically it looks quite simple. But the point is that ordinary person's wrist is undeveloped to an extent that he is not able to make at least the right angle between back of the hands and forearm. Yoga-teachers recommend a special preparatory exercise for working out the wrist apart from the wall. Stand on all fours, turn fingers back, closely press palms against the floor, and try to sit down on your heels without losing contact between palms and floor. In so doing you are required to bend wrists to opposite side till the acute angle. Of course, after that you will be able to make the right angle without any efforts and even with feeling of distinct release. It was noticed that you will need the same position of hands for mastering any type of handstand; and there are an innumerable multitude of these asanas. However not all of them are necessarily inverted postures, therefore you will start to learn them very soon.

Invariable 'Sense of Equilibrium'

Unnecessarily to struggle for cultivating sense of equilibrium since psychological demand is undeniable. In this case the border between psychic and physical abilities is essentially thin. In league of mind and body the one's weakness calls another's weakness invariably. You will feel perplexedly, if you stumble accidentally, and vice versa you stumble on level ground unless you are racked in verity of your deed and have no self-confidence. Equilibrium is a quality of consciousness, which is needed for many asanas including special group of balancing postures. We are going to explore herein nothing else than last-mentioned asanas, but don't forget that your developed sense of equilibrium will be required very often. You need to keep balance in inverted asanas, both at back and forward bends, in all kinds of combined variations (like headstand with twisting).

For performing of any balancing postures you should just slightly touch the wall controlling equilibrium or stand close to the wall to correlate body position with its surface. Formerly we marked few poses among standing asanas where you need to keep the balance. However there are a lot of standing postures on one leg which are suitable specifically for development of equilibrium as well as some sitting asanas demand of stability. All of them are mastered according to the general arrangement. Firstly you perform them against the wall; then you touch the wall with one point of the body; finally you stand apart of the wall but keep such a distance that you could easily lean on its surface in the same moment when you loose the balance. Yoga-teachers always note that the secret of equilibrium is fixed looking on any selected stationary point, and then lower the point then easier to stand without shaking.

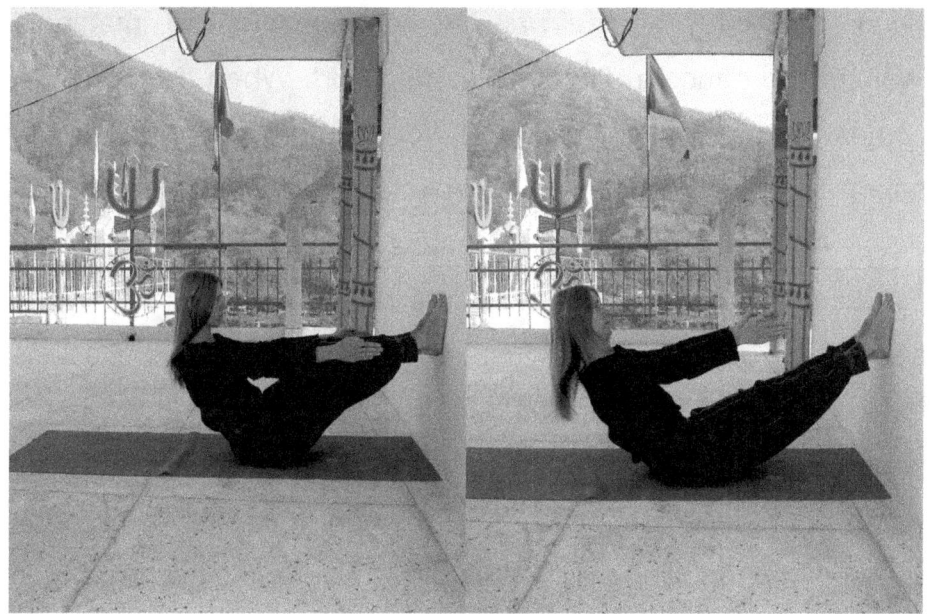

Photos 23-24

But there are some special events also: for instance, when you perform Navasana then the wall can serve as a counterbalance. Thrust your feet against the wall at the face level, keeping half-bent legs (Photo 23), and gradually straighten them pushing off the wall and removing corpus backward (Photo 24). This motion helps to produce tension, which is necessary for alignment of spine and head in slanting line. You may interlock your fingers and put the lock under the nape in order to release retention of pose. Check how the power of pushing feet against the wall is converted into the power for keeping your spine erect. You create the force in your legs and then move this force through your body up resembling the current's transfer by wire. Then try to stay off the wall but continue pushing imaginary 'wall' to reproduce in flesh the same effort. When the body becomes the erect one then it will work as the required counterbalance to legs, and you will be able to maintain equilibrium.

After you mastered Navasana apart from the wall, you can use the skill for performing the next asana. Exactly in the same way Ubhaya Padangushtasana is held by pushing legs forward. It looks very similar with Navasana though there is the only difference: you hold big toes with your fingers or put your palms on your footsteps. In that case you make the same effort to keep the equilibrium, but you push your feet against own hands instead of the wall. At the perfect stretching of straight legs, arms and spine, the whole body forms a 'triangle', which is required to be kept standing on one corner. If you have already aligned all sides and created necessarily tension inside of structure then the asana has stabilized down to the ground. Now you can face up without any difficulty and even face back (turning your head up) and close your eyes calmly. When all three sides of 'triangle' are fixed, then you can relax and allow them elongate, but your body will not shake even in the slightest degree.

Twisting: One Wall from Both Sides

The psychology of twisting is plenty ambiguous as well as the twisting itself is a paradoxical motion. Starting from psychophysiology namely twisting has the strongest effect on spinal column that is main channel of connection between brain and all the rest of your body. Nervous system in totality depends upon the condition of spinal column therefore twisting helps to make true the impaired coordination of movement, to make away with psychosomatic diseases of internals, and restore emotional security. 'Flexibility of spine means youth of body', - that statement is not unreasonable to be repeated many times, since it is really multifaceted. Symbolically twisting develops the skill to writhe oneself free or dislocate from any situation. Any twisting in asana should be mastered on both sides, and this habit works as insurance from phenomenon of kinking in all senses.

The most important is attention for division of body into upper and lower halves, which are turning to opposite directions. Commonly such position happens rarely without special efforts along with formation of volume on a broader scale. Twisting – the most extensional work in asanas, since it required turning of the body around its central axis. One would think that seeking for possibility of correlation with immobile vertical plane is unduly in this case. Nevertheless in the concrete all kinds of twisting need two actions at the same time. You should push hands to one side and thrust feet to the opposite side, and namely these movements become very easy in standing or sitting position against the wall. Although the wall is irreplaceable for mastering deep back bending and you will find more variations in the case of arching, it makes sense to perform twisting before bending. The main reason is that namely twisting but not forward bending is considered to be the basic category of poses for compensation of arching or back bending.

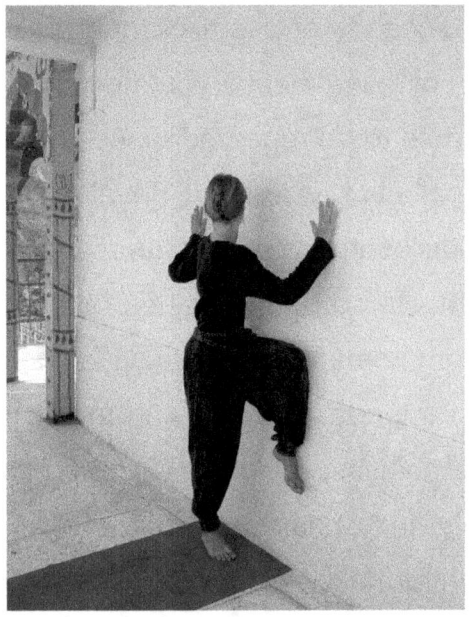

Photo 25

In standing position you can use available skills for body alignment against the wall and mastering right angles between limbs and corpus. Just now the wall is really present on one side for lower half-body and on another side for upper half-body

(Photo 25). At the very beginning you may adopt relieved version putting your footstep on some shelf, for example a low window sill. Then surely your knee will be higher and you will be able to belay elbow of the opposite arm behind this knee, thus making something like leverage for corpus turning. In this case you produce back pressure: knee is pushing elbow and simultaneously elbow is pushing knee. As a result of pressure compensation, your body is completely straight and vertical axis is not broken, however twisting becomes much stronger. But you gain the best effect in the case if you press your hand against the wall and continue pushing the same wall with the bent leg.

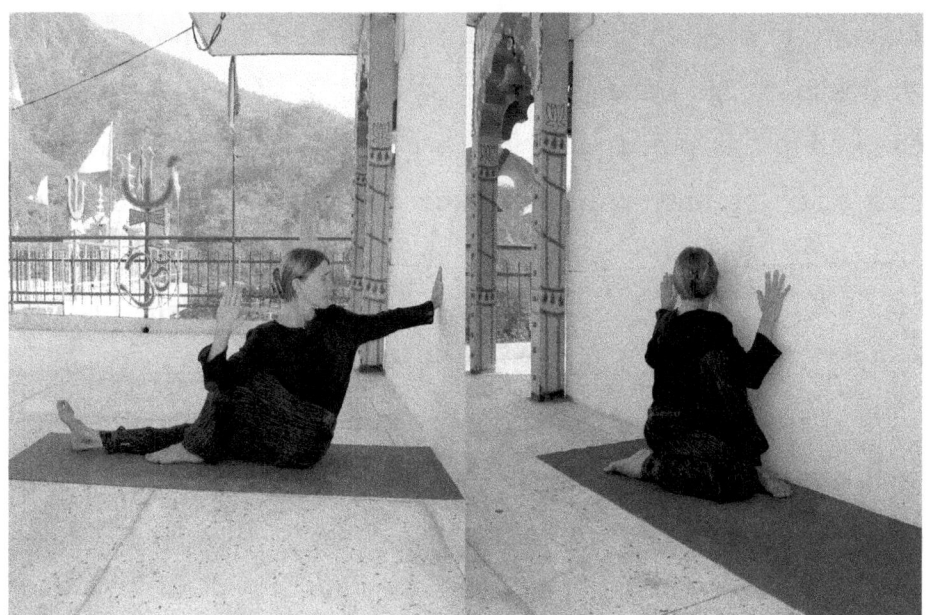

Photos 26-27

In sitting position you can use the same principle adding secondary stress from pushing another hand against the wall also (Photo 26). At that you may sit either on the floor or on the low wooden block, but be aware of different areas of pressure in your spine choosing any type of location. Moreover in the last variation (on the block) this posture becomes the balancing one to a certain degree. However the extreme twisting is available when you are sitting with side against the wall belaying outer leg back like in Virasana (Photo 27). It makes sense firstly to master this asana separately from the wall. Sit on the floor between your heels previously removing calf muscles aside with help of your hands that needless tension in knees would not be caused. Then try to deepen this posture: remove heels from hips as far as possible aside and lay down on your back between calves. Grateful to this preparation you will not worry about position of your outer leg anymore. So you can completely relax your legs and concentrate your mind on twisting of the spine column.

In both standing and sitting positions the twisting is performed with the reference to axis parallel to the wall. However if your spine is suppressed because of wrong habits then you should master twisting in lying position where your back can be relaxed and extended much easier. When you lie on you back you can utilize a thrust of footstep against the wall for fixation of the leg which is apt to move aside following to the twisting body. Try to perform at least the simplest twisting. Bend one leg and put your foot on the knee of straight leg, then put the opposite palm on the raised knee and push it against the floor. At the same time turn your head to the opposite side. In order not to bend but twist your spine, you should fix both ends of the line. Always keep your foot pressed against the wall and your shoulders close to the floor. Move your hips a little bit aside before twisting, otherwise body will fall sideways and become beveled.

In any twisting firstly you extend spine uniformly throughout the length. Then your spinal bones will not press against each other producing serious injuries. If you have any problems with your back, you should start mastering twisting in standing positions with forward bending, where the entire spine is extended and relaxed. Classical variation is the above-mentioned 'triangle', when you put the opposite hand on the floor close to the front foot, turning the whole corpus. But the most comfortable twisting is possible in forward bending with widely separated feet. Just put one hand before you at the central line and arise another hand up in the vertical. You have already learned how to master this asana with back against the wall.

Back Bending: One More Vertical

'Deep arch' is the main aspect in body's flexibility as well as the personal flexibility. Probably in the context of behavior the word 'flexibility' provokes numerous positive or negative associations in everybody's mind. Arch or back bending is far from the natural pose, as a matter of fact any common person cannot succeed even to straighten up completely and throw off an ill-

bowed back. Why the further aggravation of arching backwards is suggested? As a rule, only artists need an extreme back bending. But except the fact that unnatural behavior requires specific motivation and conscious effort, one cold-technical detail is quite remarkable. While bending forward we tried to 'form in twain' or achieve the creation of a single vertical line at combination both upper and lower body parts. But we will never succeed to construct the only vertical axis in arching or bending backwards. In order to master arching we should form two parallel vertical axes, namely separately for upper and lower body parts where legs and arms serve as prolongation.

There are a lot of variations with support of the wall for mastering of back bending. You can use the wall in the capacity of a particular vertical line, establishing two-by-two variations for development of each asana. These lines are not true vertical but rather inclined however nominally we use the ideal model that is probability bound. Moreover some arches (lying on the side) are performed entirely in the horizontal plane, although in that case we could find the vertical axis as the center of a circular arc. Also some arching asanas require beginning from the horizontal position, then forming the vertical line for one half of the body, and after converting it into the second horizontal plane above the first surface. You can observe this process mastering Bhujangasana ('cobra') and Shalabhasana ('locust'). As a result two verticals are not axes of body but they serve as the borders of 'dead space' or body's place. Nevertheless it is not our intention to deepen into geometry endlessly. We rest upon the fundamental version, namely the simplest deep back bending wherein legs and arms are vertical and parallel.

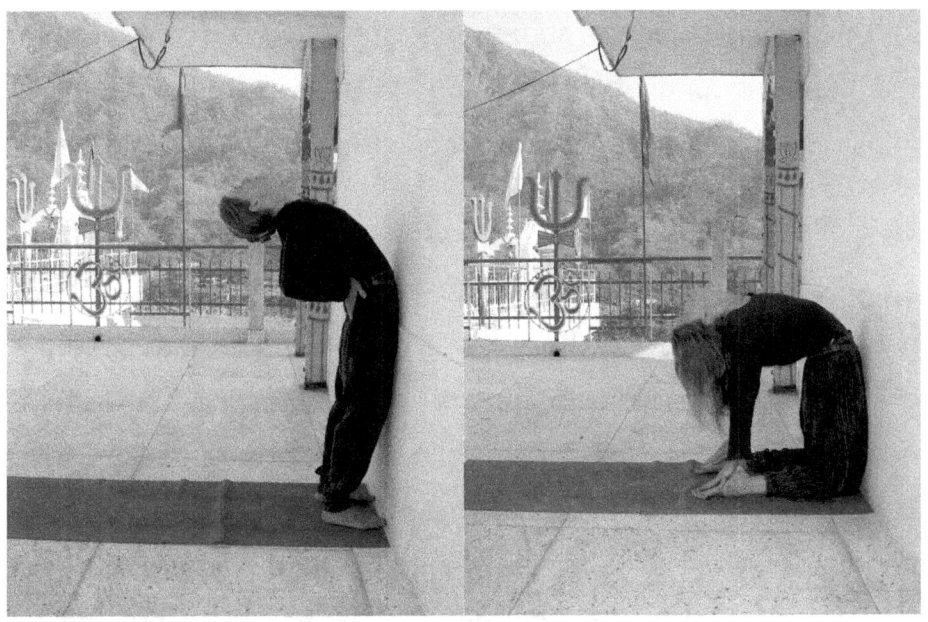

Photos 28-29

Selected type of arching can be associated with semi-inverted asanas since half-body is conversed: either upper part (in Chakrasana, 'bridge') or lower part (in Dhanurasana, 'bow'). Thus distantly we make preparations for mastery of inverted asanas against the wall. For elemental example, we can observe how to workout 'bridge' from standing posture. At the start a disciple handles along the wall, and at the limit he attempts to put down palms on the floor. In general one should be careful in back bending that spine column would be preserved from trauma, and in that case at first the wall enacts 'insurer'. When your arch will become deeper the average then you will use support of the wall in order to deepen it till 'frontier'. In the process the basic safety arrangements are extension of the spine and mainly aspiration for arching chest area rather than the small of the back, where your spine is too sensitive for a break.

Preparation: Simple Retroversion

The simplest variation of arching in standing position lies in the fact that you decline all over backwards. In that case the wall's function is similar to the limit stop at bending foreword. In the same way the wall doesn't allow your legs to decline from the vertical line and it lets to concentrate on your back. Try to stand facing the wall, strongly press your thighs against the vertical surface, further abut your heels of the hands on the small of the back turning fingers downward, and then recede (Photo 28). Herewith continue to pull your head with top upwards without overturning back. Since your thighs are pressed against the wall, it is not difficult to work with your arms in order to extend your spine throughout the length flexing it uniformly in circular arc with the exception of any breaks. It is essential to bring your elbows together till the shoulders' width that hands' thrust would become stronger. The same force helps to keep your head in the line with the spine, because the deeper back bending the harder neck stretching. The head should not fall backward but you should decline your neck with a controlled motion continuing the circular arc of the spine. It's easer if previously you put your footsteps not together but on shoulders' breadth.

Now you may proceed to performance of classical Ushtrasana ('camel') against the wall (Photo 29). This is the same posture merely you stand on the knees and thrust your palms against footsteps. You can start to perform the asana in two opposite ways. In one case you are standing on the knees and reaching your footsteps with your hands. In another case you are sitting on the heels and raising your thighs up to the stop against the wall. The last version seems easier since you can base yourself upon arms stronger. You should start from sitting position and further you can master the standing position. Really the order depends on your abilities. If you have developed good arching but still you have week muscles of arms and back then you are able to relax in Ushtrasana without any problems. But if you have stiff back and strong arms, then you should start from a little declining in standing position. Suffering from stiffness you are not allowed to hurry up throwing back your head. It's better to continue looking forward for a long enough not to hurt your neck. Gradually the entire back will get over a new condition, and you will be able to workout cervical spine specially.

Paradoxical 'Arching in Bending'

Reasonably large number of asanas demands that body assumes paradoxical position 'arch in bend'. You can prepare to it's performing against the wall too, where you can relax completely and influence namely the thoracic area. According to Yoga therapy this pose is suitable for all officials who spread whole day in their office poking their heads over computer's keyboard or 'security papers'. These postures are good enough in order to relax thoracic girdles, open thoracic cage to the limit, and unbend body to the opposite direction. In this connection the small of the back becomes relaxed too, though it's bent back also. But this arching is entirely within limits of your operational capabilities, and you can be sure that you will not overreach yourselves.

Stand with your face against the wall at intervals of about one step but take into account that depending on a distance the main pressure will fall on different parts of spinal column. It is a good idea to change the distance according to your conditions. Anyway your legs stay in the vertical position always. Put palms on the wall as high as possible then sag all over, slipping with palms of straitened arms alone the wall as low as possible (Photo 30). Try to touch the wall by the central point of your chest, though it can stay in some distance also. If you are able to feel the whole body then this movement looks like the effort to move legs and arms meet halfway, but on parallel vertical lines. Your tail bone is pulling up similar to 'dog' posture and other bends, and the highest point of the chest is going down similar to 'bridge' posture and other arches (though in introverted view). As a result we attain the paradoxical 'arch in bend'.

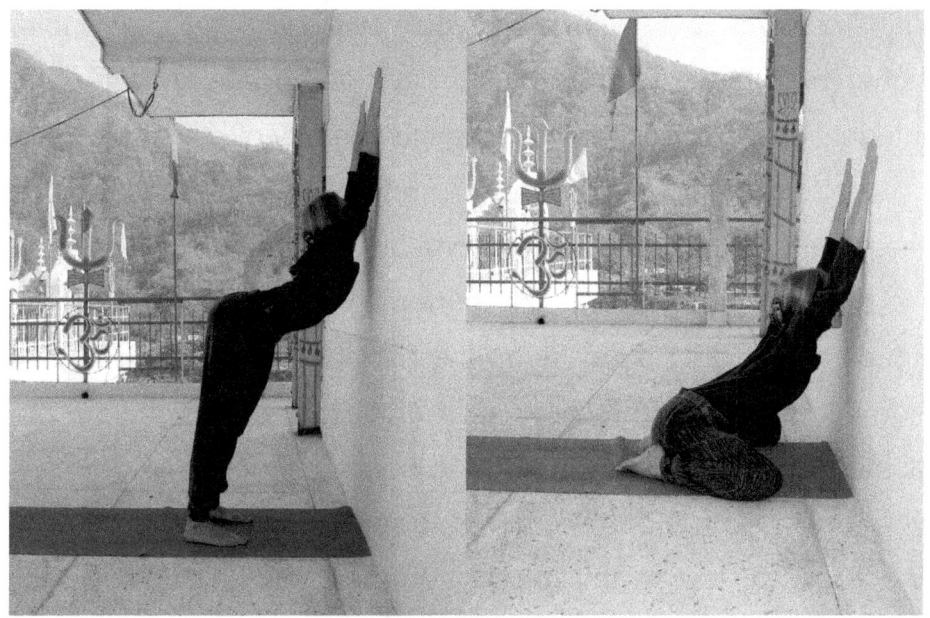

Photos 30-31

In order to force to work out the small of the back you can master the posture in sitting position (Photo 31). Sit on your knees in front of the wall in some distance, perform the above-mentioned Virasana, and separate your knees as wide as possible that space before abdomen would be free. Then repeat the previous motion of arms and back but in this case pulling not only your chest to the wall but also the abdomen to the floor. In such position you work for simultaneous opening of chest and hips. Like before you should check the distance from the wall, since if you are sitting far then your small of the back is arching, but if you are sitting close then your thoracic area is arching. As usually anyway it is better to apportion the arching along your spinal column evenly, feeling your own back on the whole, rather than give attention to the each patch alternatively. The integrity of consciousness causes the integrity of physical form.

If you need to prepare for performing of this movement, then you can do the same exercise as you did before for twisting. Move over from the wall, perform Virasana sitting on your knees and putting buttocks on the floor between feet. However now you should separate knees in order to lie down on your abdomen while before you separated heels in order to lie down on your back. At that be careful not to remove your buttocks from the floor, otherwise this type of preparation loses its significance. If your buttocks start to rise up then it's better to push them on the same place and stay orphan in semi-bending, waiting till your ligaments will become stretched. With this objection in mind you may base yourselves upon elbows to relax your groin. Thus you are limited to bending without arching while your body habituates to a new position. Coming back to the wall, you will be able to concentrate on arching stronger.

Standard 'Trine' of Arches

Now it makes sense that you proceed to work out the trine of classical back-bending asanas such as Bhujangasana ('cobra'), Shalabhasana ('locust') and Dhanurasana ('bow'). All together these three postures exert integrated arching effect. 'Bow' is symmetrical to 'bridge' but much easier because you need less force in order to rise up limbs than all the body. The upper part of spine is bending in 'cobra', the lower part of spine is bending in 'locust', and both arches are combined in 'bow' where main pressure falls on the middle part of spine. There aren't many options for mastering 'cobra' with support of the wall, since really bending is essential when you start declining back from the vertical line. First you can try a similar pose 'up-facing dog', Urdhva Mukha Shvanasana (Photo 32), where wall serves for control only, and you can check yourself with touching the wall by progressively lower point of your chest. The same situation is happening with 'bow' (Photo 33), where the thrust knees against the wall is convenient at the floor level. Further you need to stay off wall and catch your ankles with hands.

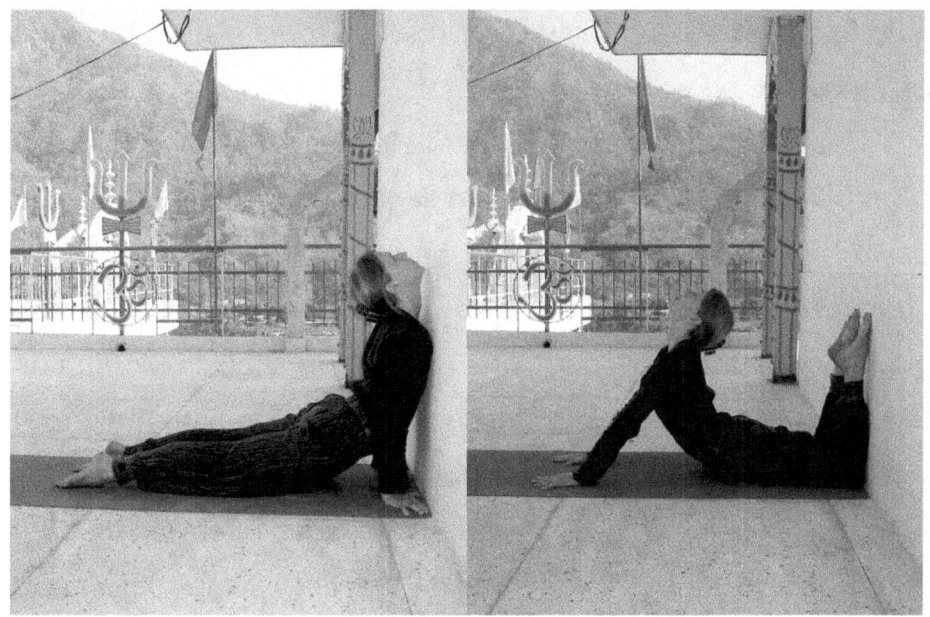

Photos 32-33

At the limit the 'locust' is pushed through Viparita Shalabhasana or 'chin stand', and in that case you can use the support of the wall for quite a long time. In standard variation you don't just arise legs above the floor but move them with a whisk upwards to vertical position, and then even put them beyond the head on the floor. Firstly you should master arch standing on the knees with your chin lowered on the floor and arms stretched forward. When you relax thoracic spine you should reach to put your neck and upper chest on the floor. You would better start to perform this asana against the wall also: turn with your head off from the wall you can gradually creep upwards with your legs and abdomen. In addition it is necessary always to touch the floor with your chest, stretch your legs as high as possible, and relax your thoracic spine. After mastering arch against the wall you may try to raise legs with a whisk.

If you prefer to be limited to simplest variation of 'locust' (Photo 34), then perform the next series of movements. First lie down on your stomach pressing your knees against the wall that your calves would be oriented upwards alone the wall. Then put your palms similar to 'cobra' that means you should put them on the floor on both sides of the body at the breast's height. It makes sense to keep hands in this position from the very beginning that you could control your movement. Push against the floor compensates pressure on the cervical spine, which can become too strong for you at the start. After that press your toes against the wall and try to straighten your legs removing them from the wall. Little by little you will be able to shift from one foot to another one upwards alone the wall. At the same time you will move your corpus closer to the wall, deepening arch.

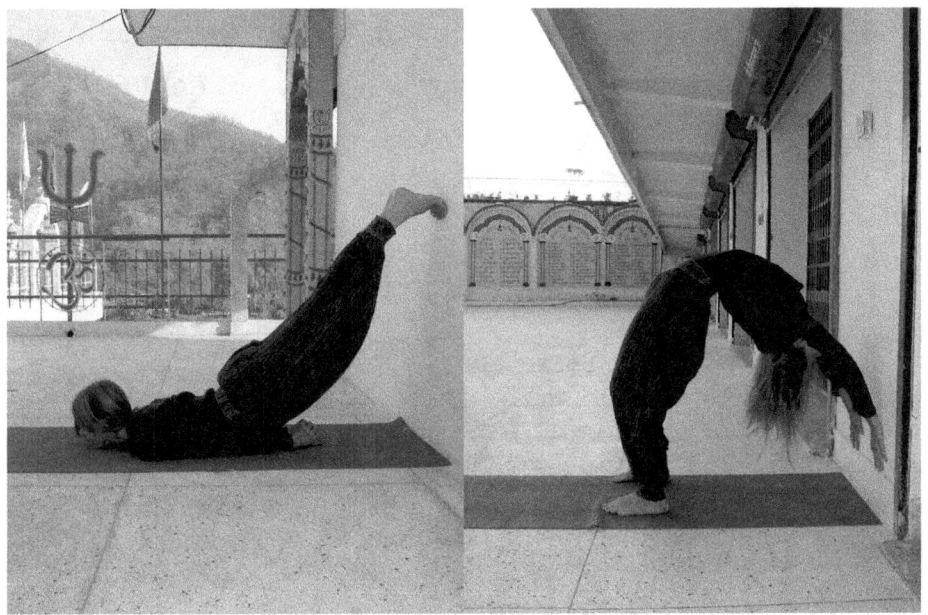

Photos 34-35

When you come back to original position and don't change location, then you get remarkable possibility for immediate performing of 'cobra' similar to 'bow' according to its shape in this case. Staying in the original pose you can ask somebody to stand with his feet on the small of your back. One can mill about, properly kneading with his heels your spine in the state of little arching. In order to feel more comfortable at the process of such "hard" massage you can put under your pubic bone something like folded blanket. In prospect at your own will you may alternate the lifts of lower and upper body resting in each next posture after the previous one. Thus you workout every part of your back carefully as if moving the wave of arching through your spine bottom-upwards and return. If you will be able to find a proper rhythm for such alteration then you will get the excellent dynamical sequence of asanas or vinyasa in yogic dialect.

'Bridge' – Arch as Such

Truly there is no better support for mastering Urdha Dhanurasana ('bridge') at the very beginning, than the wall's prop. A lot of variations are invented that the wall would be used suitably namely for performing of this asana. As you know, it is possible to perform 'bridge' starting from lying or standing positions; and definitely the first way is much easier then the second one. Now let us give consideration to the first variation, where the wall is adopted according to our working habit, though in inverted perspective in comparison with the above-described triad of asanas. Precisely you should set up your palms behind your head pressing the heels of the hands against the wall before performing the 'bridge'. Needless to say, your fingers are turned from the wall to the body. Stretching your limbs and perform the pose as good as possible at the moment you should start mastering it in details. Try to straiten your arms completely and bring elbows together, then push the floor with your legs (also make them as straight as possible), and establish your arms in the vertical line. At the same time you should pull your chest to the wall; now it becomes obviously that you mastered this movement standing against the wall at first attempts of arching.

This posture has many other variations in dependence on hands' location and different props especially wooden blocks. They are useful for support; however you can get options for making life complicated with their help. We can notice among them some details in position of straight arms, which is oriented at the limit to performing of handstand. Advanced practitioners master Urdha Dhanurasana till such degree that they choose not Tadasana (stand) but Hasta Vrikshasana (handstand) as the next pose accepting it as original position also. They start from handstand, perform 'bridge' and come back to handstand. Even if you are far from the inspiration by similar 'wire dancing' then you should be aware how to use the criterion for correction of thoracic girdle. For this purpose it's enough to do at least inner movement by arms' muscles to keep elbows apart from the wall and at the same time press armpits against the wall. In this case an outward visibility of the result is not more important then the correct intention of effort.

Now let us proceed to observe variations. First of all you can put your palms not on the floor close to the wall but directly on the wall leaning the tips of the middle fingers against the floor. If the surface of the wall is not slippery, then you can put your palms on the wall in the same position though a little bit above the floor (Photo 35). In that case back arch will be not very deep, and your body will get chance to form a habit to understand at its physical level what is going on. Further you can put your hands on wooden blocks moved up against the wall; for sure it will make your task easier in the initial stage. However in the opposite way if you wish to deepen even without that excellent arch, then you can put your palms on the floor just before blocks. At the same time you should continue pulling your chest to the wall inclining your straight arms towards the wall. It is possible to perform these motions without any wall working out with legs only. But in default of distinct criterion in the form of wall you can get the false impression about an arching degree.

If the distance between your chest and the wall is too large, then you can use blocks otherwise. Accept the most approachable position and ask somebody to put block between your chest and the wall. Push your legs that you keep block bearing heavily thereupon with your chest. However don't arise your chest up, just the opposite, pull your pubic bone up. In other words herein you will gain something grateful to arch in the small of back. But you are able to control the arching only in the case, if you move your corpus forward without arising it. Nevertheless you should tend to bend basically in the thoracic spine, while the lower part of your back is arching in the minimal degree and only because of complete relaxation and stretching.

The most therapeutically variation of Urdha Dhanurasana is hanging from a beam, usual stool or chair with the completely relaxed body. Seat on the stool facing the wall in such distance, that you could straighten your legs and lean your feet against the floor or the wall just above the floor. Then slowly recline your body and retract your straight arms. If possible you can put your palms on the floor and perform Urdha Dhanurasana uplifting your body above the stool and again coming back on the support in order to relax in arching. There are two important moments: firstly, performing posture you should control position of your head avoiding any break in the neck area; secondly, finishing the posture you should arise up your arching chest. But never try to bend and pull your head forward before your chest. Fulfillment of both conditions is very essential to protect your neck from any type of injury.

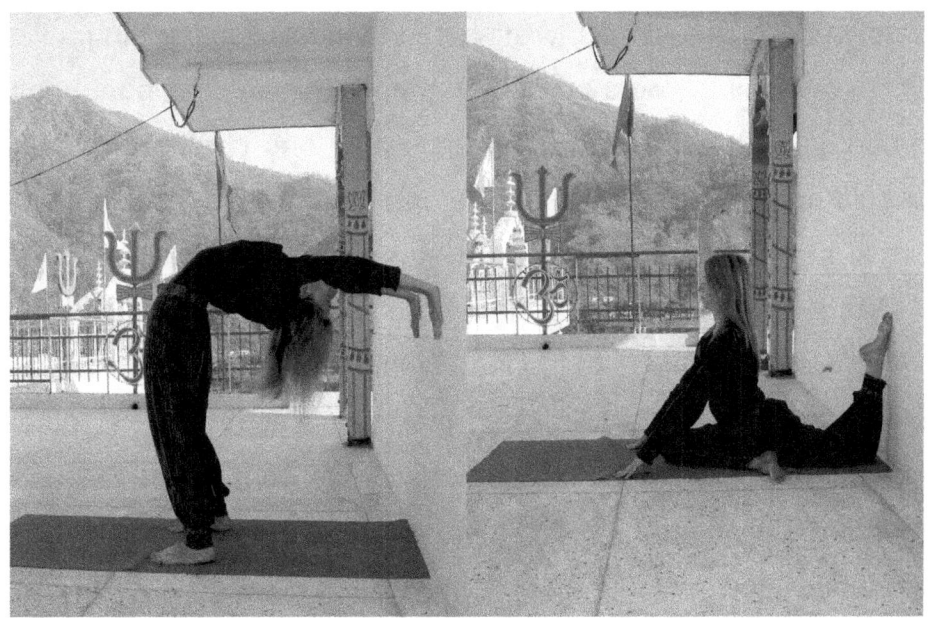

Photos 36-37

Then you can master an input from the standing position to Urdha Dranurasana and an output to the original pose with the support of the wall (Photo 36). At the same time you can start working out the opposite movement namely an output from Urdha Dhanurasana to handstand and the following input to the standing position with feet on the floor. Firstly this movement is performed against the wall also. It is remarkable that if you have well-developed shoulders' joints, then an output from 'bridge' through handstand becomes even easier than the common output from 'bridge' to Tadasana. In both cases you gradually handle on the wall with your limbs. Respectively you should turn with your head or legs against the wall. Don't forget about the contra-pose after finishing back bending exercises: first you must perform any simple twisting and then forward bending.

As well it would be useful to consider an individual body proportions. If you have short limbs and long corpus then you should not hurry up to master the output from "bridge" to legs or arms. In that case it is necessary to workout the basic posture insistently for a long time striving to move alternatively either hands to feet or feet to hands. When in Urdha Dhanurasana hands are moving to feet, then the lower sacral part of spinal column is opening in a great measure; on the contrary, when feet are moving to hands, then the upper thoracic spine is stretching powerfully. Remember this general rule and always alternate the approach of hands and feet by some means. After getting an ability to straighten your arms in 'bridge' without any problem and keep the posture in the relaxed state, you should try to straighten your legs too. If it will become successful also, then you may master the output from 'bridge' to the standing position on your feet or palms. At the start you can use support of the wall, but soon the need of help will be abandoned.

Arch on Asymmetrical Base

Until now the question was the arch at keeping both legs in the same position being either together or at shoulders' width. The 'arch in bend' performing in the sitting position required the complete opening of hips but still its symmetry was preserved. However an arching can be added to many postures where legs are opened asymmetrically. It's possible up to and including the arch in backward forward split, when you turn your forehead up and backward till joining with the foot of the bent hind leg. Of course, this is the extreme arch; and it is strongly not recommended that beginners would try to workout something similar. Extremity is absolutely not necessarily in asanas, though the very principles of movement should be assimilated perfectly. We are going to explore such positions where arch is adumbrated. Firstly it will be difficult to understand how these poses could be included into this chapter. Nevertheless the tendency for arching is clearly represented in each asana. It is a matter of visible degree which you will be able to reach in your own practice.

The simplest overpass to an asymmetrical position is starting from 'cobra' with both calves against the wall which you have already learned. Now you should to move foreword one of your legs (Photo 37). Then you need to align whole body in vertical keeping a check on the evenness of your hips which should not be warped. Be aware that one leg would be oriented directly backward and another leg would be oriented directly forward. As may be required you should underlay a blanket below your buttocks, but in no circumstances you should not allow to fall sideways. Commonly Yoga teachers use yet band by the next way. Fix the ply of one free end at your foot, belay both hands behind your head, pull another free end, and move your hands closer to your foot till you will be able to catch your toes with your fingers. However you can use the band in the only case if your body is completely stable. You see, you need to remove both hands from the floor keeping the balance mostly on the side of the bent front leg. Otherwise you can deepen arch without any band, just displacing your palms from the floor to the front knee and slowly moving them alone your thigh as close to the corpus as possible. You may bend your arms a little bit at the movement and then gradually straighten them reclining your body back.

Hereafter you can try to repeat the same with the erect front leg. Stand with your back against the wall, bend one leg (Photo 38) and carefully move the skid foot forward slipping on the floor simultaneously lowing the back knee down till the floor level (Photo 39). Be aware that your front leg must be erect even if the distance between the perineum and the floor is still not so very small. As in the previous case, use a folded blanket or heavier bead in dependence on the size of space between body and the floor. At that you don't forget to press your calf against the wall in order to align your hips. For checking you can recall the position of your hips in the common Tadasana. Stretching up your spine you can arise both straight arms too, at the same time pulling the upper body upwards and putting the lower body downwards. After all the others you can try to decline slowly in an arc backwards to the wall. Doesn't matter, what arching extent will be succeeded.

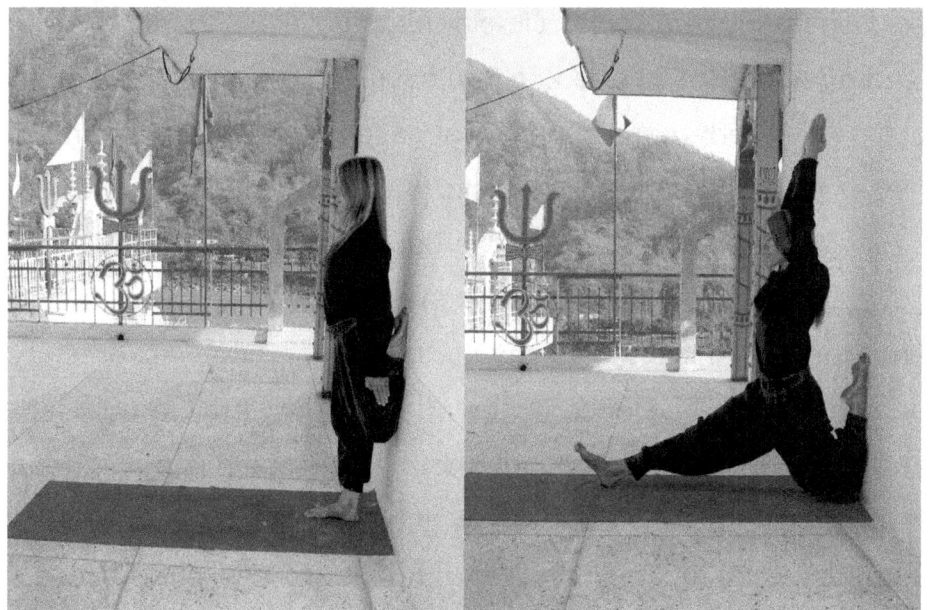

Photos 38-39

Inverted Asanas close to Wall

Perhaps body's inversion in the space exactly to the opposite position causes the strongest psycho-energy influence. It is not accidental that usually headstand is performed in the very end of the practice, just before relaxation in Shavasana. Avoiding description of all mystical effects let us observe the most obvious fact: the inversion of the whole world outlook; the exchange of point of view in the opposite way. Merely headstand allows us to look at the world alternatively, to see everything in unaccustomed perspective. In the best case the result is 'stopping of the world' or 'breaking of self-reflection's mirror'. At the same action in yogic system we expect momentary Samadhi, if instant concentration let us to catch a glimpse of the pure consciousness. Even more simple asanas like Viparita Karani Mudra (symbol of inverted action) cause reversion of the stream of time. Similarly 'candle' or Sarvangasana (posture for all limbs) makes possible to aware a holistic perception of the entire body.

Metaphors are endless around here therefore let's get down to business. It needs no explanation that the wall is suitable for the mastering of inverted asanas, since an ordinary person has no developed sense of equilibrium to perform headstand without any preparation. Though handstand is by far not a solitary posture of this sort, anyway even more stable poses require the vertical alignment. In Iyengar-style and other schools of Yoga practice there are different sequences for the mastering of Halasana ('plough'), Sarvangasana ('candle') and Vrishchicasana ('scorpion') starting from the original position with your face or back against the wall. You can develop some alternative approaches except of the simplest headstand and handstand with the support of the wall. There are postures with different locations of your palms in handstand, where it is quite difficult to keep the balance. At the same time these variations let to work-out the thoracic girdle and the thoracic spine very intensively.

'Half-Bridge' – at Approaches to Overturn

Even if you are afraid looking at any inverted asana, you should make no question of the next simple posture which is available for everyone. Lay down on your back with your legs close to the wall in such a distance that you could bend them and put feet on the wall making the right angle between calves and the vertical surface (Photo 40). Without displacing your feet and shoulders you should push your legs against the wall and arch your body upwards removing your buttocks and back from the floor. Then put your palms under the shoulder blades, bring your elbows together (till the shoulders' breadth), and relax as much as possible. Depending on your condition you can make the task easier or harder. If you are not able to raise your body up, then you may use the help of hands from the very begin-ning. Alternatively if you are able to keep arching body without hands' support, then you have to interlock your fingers and put straight arms on the floor (Photo 41). In that case you get possi-bility of stronger arching and stretching of the whole body owing to thrust with your arms against the floor and simultaneous thrust with your feet against the wall. Otherwise you can move your feet upper alone the wall, straightening the arch but then approaching the vertical inverted position. However be aware of your neck that pressing would not become too excessive.

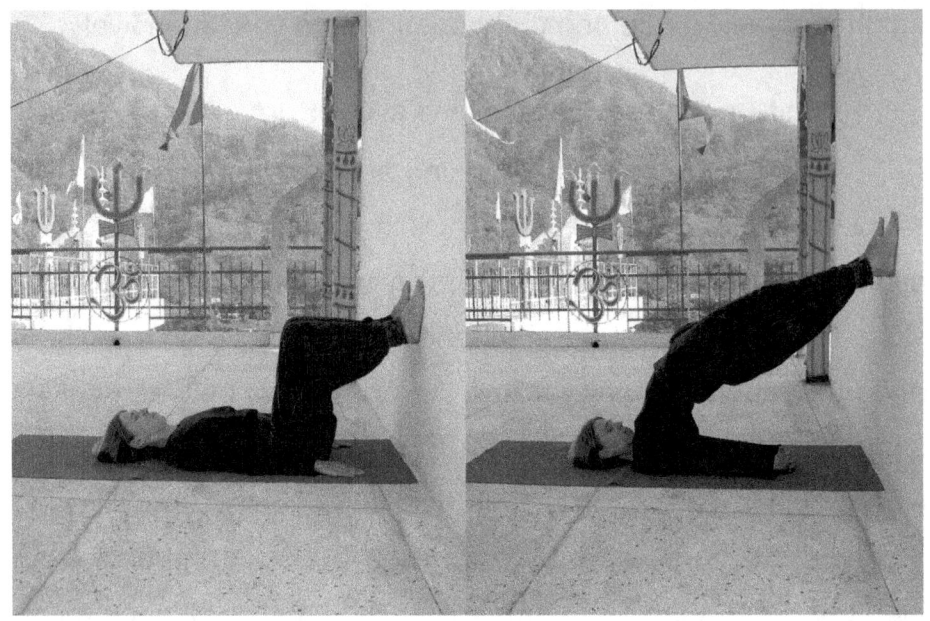

Photos 40-41

In this posture against the wall the form of your body is similar to another asana namely Setu Bandha Sarvangasana. You see that you need a deeper arch for performing of the next asana but at the same time you need not to raise your legs and there is no inverted position here. In dependence on your state at the moment the one of mentioned postures will be the preparation for another one. Simple Setu Bandha is performing in the following manner. Lie down on your back, bend your legs and put your feet close to your hips at the shoulders' breadth.

Stretch your arms alone the body and then bend them in elbows' joints. Without displacing upper arms you should establish forearms perpendicularly of the floor. Double fists, press your elbows and feet against the floor, raise your hips above the floor in one movement, and arch your whole body as high as possible. Eventually your forearms and calves became perpendicular to the floor and parallel to each other. In other words, your knees are located directly above your heels, while your fists are located directly above your elbows. It is essential that upraise would be done not by unbending legs in knees' joints but by pressing on the feet especially on their inner part. If you got tired then you can put your palms under the small of your back 'hanging' all body weight on your arms and completely relaxing. It is equally true that also you can straighten your legs forward slipping with your feet on the floor. In that case you will master the desired variation that is Setu Bandha Sarvangasana.

Halasana, Sarvangasana, Shirshasana

Let us proceed to well-known inverted asanas Halasana ('plough'), Sarvangasana ('candle'), Shirshasana (headstand). It makes sense to master these poses namely in the mentioned order, though Sarvangasana can be easier than Halasana in the case if you are not flexible enough. However you will not have problems of this sort after successful performing of forward bending. This triad is included into many sequences even for beginners, while advanced inverted asanas are unwell-known;

and ordinary people consider them the out-of-limit ones. Nevertheless the wall's support lets you start their mastering together with basic inverted postures. That is why we will describe elbow-stand and handstand underneath, when you will be preliminarily prepared after performing shoulder-stand and headstand.

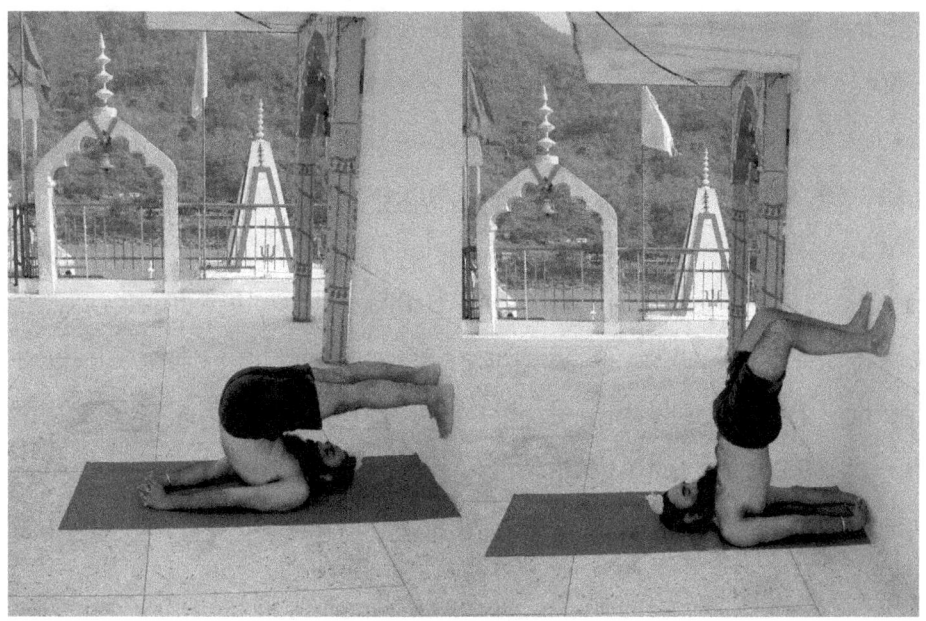

Photos 42-43

As for 'plough' the situation is quite simple since usually the main difficulty is caused by effort to bend body till such a degree that one could put toes on the floor. Therefore first you should put your feet on the wall at the available for you level above the floor (Photo 42). It is strongly recommended that you would not correct the shoulders' position when all body weight is pressing on the thoracic girdle. Otherwise you carry a risk to 'twist neck'; be aware that the same regards to all other inverted asanas too. You should admeasure the distance from the wall in advance sitting on the floor and straightening your legs that your feet would touch the wall. After making a note of your sitting place you should turn with your back against the wall and put your shoulders there. In Halasana the body must be at the right angle to the floor, therefore you will get directly the required distance after placing your feet on the wall.

For the performing of Sarvangasana the order of movements starts from the distance's checking also. Lie down on your back and press your buttocks against the wall stretching erect legs upwards in the vertical line. Some teachers recommend putting any folded blanket under the back, that your head would be lying on the floor a little bit lower than the corpus. In that case you can be sure that all the weight will be pressed on your shoulders only, while your neck will be free and relaxed. It is essential for beginners, but progressing in practice you should remove any blankets as soon as possible. Now you have a strong mind to a habitual movement: press you feet against the wall and raise an entire body till strictly vertical line that your calves become parallel to the floor (Photo 43). Then put your palms under the shoulders' blade and move your feet upwards too in the course of your body. The whole body should be in one and the same straight line from shoulders to feet.

When simple inverted asanas don't cause difficulties,

then headstand is worked out because it required more advanced sense of the equilibrium. As in other inverted asanas you should not produce superfluous pressure on your neck, therefore you must learn the correct position of hands that almost all body weight is pressed on the arms. Sit down on your knees; put your forearms on the floor, interlock your elbows (put your palms on opposite elbows crosswise) in order to find out a proper distance between elbows. Fixing your elbows on the floor you should interlock your fingers and make 'triangle' as a base for headstand. Now put your top on the floor between your palms rising your hips up. Then remove your knees from the floor, place your feet as close to the head as possible, and raise erect legs up in one smooth movement. If your prelum abdominal is not strong enough, in that case firstly you may raise bent legs, then straighten corpus up, and stretch your legs upwards.

At the start you should workout everything with your back against the wall (Photo 44), because the backward downfall is the touchiest point. Accident's prevention provides two ways how to avoid trauma losing balance apart from the wall. If you are flexible then you just put your feet on the floor behind your head. Otherwise you should round your back quickly and roll over your head. When you use support of the wall then you can remove from its surface alternatively one and another leg and eventually both legs together. The alignment of your body must be exactly equal to Tadasana, what we mentioned at the very beginning. In order to relax your neck in more degree you can ask somebody to put a wooden block between your back and the wall at shoulders' blade level. Make effort to keep the block at the same place pushing elbows against the floor. This trick can help you to remove pressure from your neck, though you should master the proper work by your hands anyway.

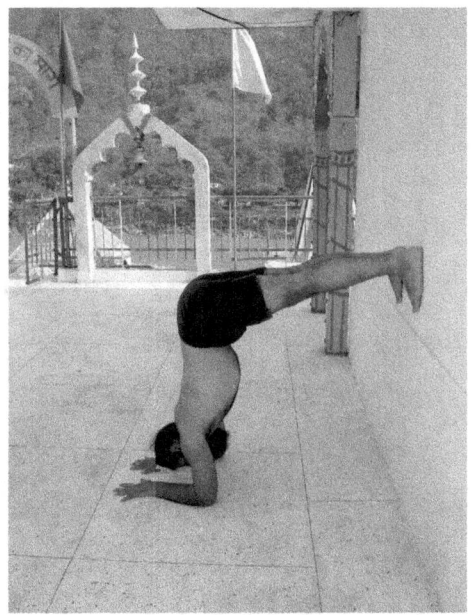

Photo 44

Also the wall's support is useful for the mastering of the output from headstand with erect legs including such intermediate asana as Urdhva Dhanurasana. This is nothing else than simple holding of legs at the right angle to corpus. You can be located with your back against the wall that your hips would not move behind your head. Another option lies in the fact that you perform Shirshasana with your face against the wall, from the start placing your head in straight legs' distance from the wall. While moving your legs down till horizontal level you can put your feet on the wall and workout the right angle between legs and corpus being in more relaxed condition. Moreover you will get a distinct criterion of the vertical line. This position is useful for the preparation to perform Pincha Mayurasana. However it is not headstand but forearms stand, and your head is hanged in suspension above the floor.

Forearm Balance

Better if you start mastering forearms' balance with your face against the wall. Admeasure a distance from the wall to be equal to the length of your legs and find a place for the establishing your elbows by the renowned method. As a preliminary you can squeeze a wooden block between your palms. It will help you to keep forearms in parallel lines on the floor for better stability. In the advanced version you can set up your elbows as for headstand and joint your palms together. Then base yourselves upon forearms and walk with your feet upwards on the wall while your body will accept the next form (Photo 45). All body and upper arms are in line, your head is hanging freely between your arms, and erect legs are parallel to the floor pressing feet against the wall. Then move your feet on the wall as high as possible, otherwise try to remove your feet from the wall and push your legs up one by one or simultaneously.

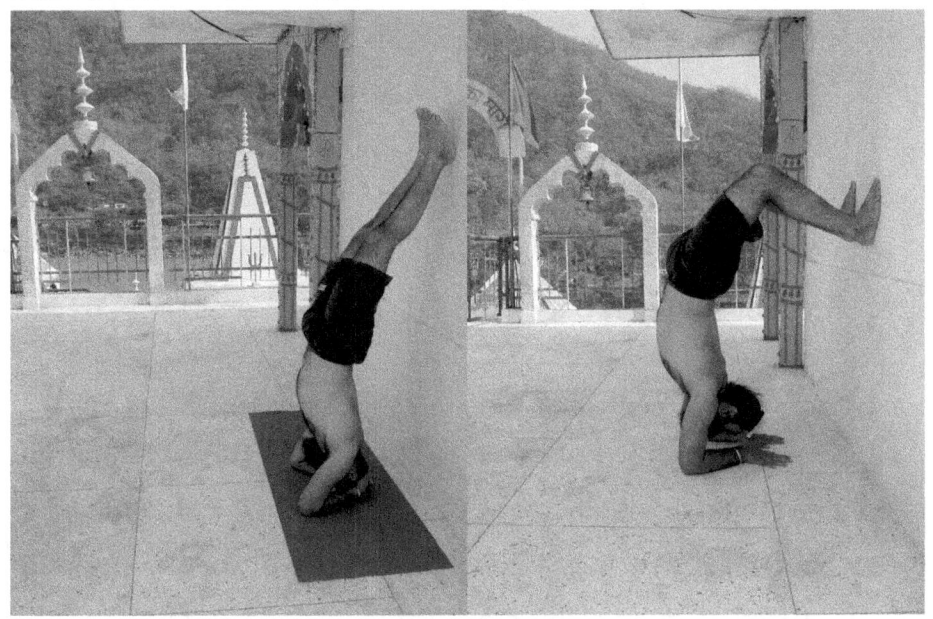

Photos 45-46

It is more difficult but more beneficial if you start mastering Pincha Mayurasana with your back against the wall (Photo
46). Establish your forearms on the floor in such a way that tips
of your fingers would almost touch the wall. Your elbows should
be in calves' length from the wall, but usually calves are little bit
longer than forearms. Then put your feet on the wall bending
legs in knees' joints, and your calves will become at the right
angle with your thighs. Now you can try to raise your legs up in
the vertical and put feet back on the wall alternatively. In the
same way you can move your feet upwards alone the wall
slowly straightening your legs and little arching your back. If still
you are using a block, you can try to perform this asana turning

your forearms in such a manner that your palms would be facing upwards. Shoulders' opening and neck's relaxation are much easier in this position. Moreover you can try to pull your head to the wall in order to open your shoulders' blade that you could erect your back completely. After mastering the position with erect legs you can add back arching, but very carefully.

Hand Balance

Behold we have already got to the last basic asana and soon you may completely relax your whole body without leaving the wall. The question is handstand, and we noticed few elements in simple asanas during our practical guidance that you would be prepared to perform this task. If you have weak arms and legs then you should learn this posture with your face against the wall. In that case there is no need to push feet against the floor strongly to bring the body's weight on your arms by one motion. It is enough to move you feet alone the wall bottom-upwards till you will get the highest point which is available for you at the moment. However there is an essential fault of this control theory because it is quite difficult to put palms close to the wall from the very beginning, and as a result your body will be reclined even after full stretching. Maybe you are able to move your palms closer to the wall after performing handstand, but it is not for sure with your weak arms. Otherwise you would perform handstand with your back against the wall from the very beginning. But the reclined posture is good enough that you could feel the work of your body in this position.

In order to perform handstand with your back against the wall (Photo 47), you can ask for a help according to some rules. One of options is the following. Your assistant stands with his back against the wall spreading his feet at shoulders' breadth. You should come closer, bend down and fix your palms between his feet pressing your elbows against his knees. Then he takes your hips and rise your body up, and at the same time you push your feet against the floor that move them upwards in one movement. An assistant needs to remove his head aside in time that you would not beat his face with your feet, but anyway he will do it instinctively. Next he should proceed to pull your thighs up stretching your body, while you press your palms against the floor with the same intention.

Thus you will learn to work with your arms in handstand, and you don't use your arms as support only. Constantly you try to stretch your body in line as high as possible; and at the process you eliminate arching of your back and open your shoulders. We noted one version of preparing your shoulders for handstand that is the performing of 'down facing dog' with support of your palms or forearms. Any Iyengar-teacher can show the way how to make this posture more complicated: you should squeeze a wooden block between your palms and tie up your upper arms by a band till your shoulders' breadth. You can use this construction just for mastering of handstand if in good time you prepare the ply measuring it along the length of your forearm from elbow to a cavity between thumb and finger. Then you need to put this ply around your upper arms a little bit higher than elbows. One more criterion is the location of the band just above your top when you raise your arms up keeping your head directly between upper arms. Of course, it is much better if you learn to feel your own body instead of any blocks and bands.

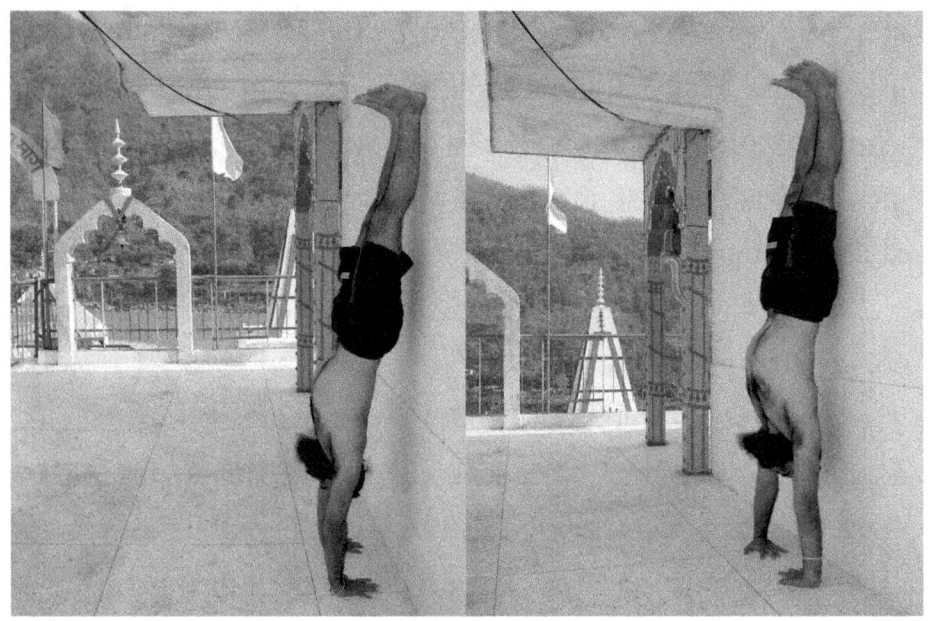

Photos 47-48

Becoming accustomed to the common handstand you may proceed to mastering of different variations even if you are not able to remove feet from the wall at least for few seconds. Above all from the very outset you should workout the posture correctly while the sense of the equilibrium will be developed in the course of time since it requires prolonged reorganization in brain's functions. Merely you should force your body to perform an inverted position every day doing unwearying efforts to master handstand; and sooner or later the result will be got by itself. As for the concrete variations you can try to put your palms on the floor in different ways: either turning your fingers inside (Photo 48) or turning them backwards and outwards. You can find all these poses in the second sequence of ashtanga Vinyasa Yoga too. In the first instance it makes sense to work out all prenominate hand positions in 'down facing dog' and then in handstand. You need strong arms for performing these variations otherwise you take risks to smash your head against floor.

When you find yourselves absolutely steadily then you can complicate the issue of performing handstand putting your palms not on the floor but on any stable support. In that case the task itself will require becoming stronger and more perfect in performing of each motion otherwise nothing will happen. For sure the suggested complication intends not to overpass to acrobatics, but to grind the technique of the asana. You see, you will not be able to do careless work anymore and raise legs up one after another one pushing with the strongest leg. If you put your palms on some platform then you must push with both legs definitely. So you should be able to straighten your legs in one controlled movement just in-flight from the floor to the wall. Obviously this innovation is comparable with the performing of headstand raising erect legs up.

Eventually you can workout different positions of your legs and corpus. The simplest option is Bhadrasana in handstand. Firstly try to feel the posture lying down with your back on the floor. Stretch your body in line, bend your legs, joint your feet together pulling them close to perineum, and open your thighs in order to put knees on the floor on both sides. In the process your back should be pressed against the floor as well as against the wall in the real handstand. After mastering this pose you can try to perform 'lotus' in handstand, of course if you are able to do Padmasana without any help of your hands. In that case performing Bhadrasana you should press the small of your back against the wall and one by one move your feet above your thighs. I testify that many practitioners including centenarian elders do everything the above-described easily. Moreover there is nothing more impressive than 'scorpion' where handstand is combined with such a deep arch that yogi puts his feet on his shoulders. As for all arches you can move your feet step by step downwards alone the wall, simultaneously rising your head upwards for the equilibrium...

Nevertheless even the bare listing can produce an abnormal stress at the start; therefore let us improve relaxation skills. It is essential since the more complicated asana is performed the more perfect ability for deep relaxation is required. Otherwise your practice is accompanied by traumatism. Proper allowance must be made that quoted below technique of relaxation is beneficial after standing and bending asanas mostly. But it is unnecessarily and even contraindicative after performing of any inverted asanas. The reason is not far to seek. You kept the legs above the head long enough, therefore now it would be better if you would straight them horizontally on the floor.

Relaxation with Legs on Wall

Relaxation is the highlight of the performance in any psychotherapy session. Nowadays people are bent on means for relaxation no less than on means for exaltation. Thereat, the relaxation is not the end in itself but rather a method to get a comfort and forget oneself like an innocent hypnotic or narcotic. Paradoxically in order to relax modern people use namely an extreme excitement whereupon the leisure industry is built. What actually a person needs if not the passing mental alienation at any price. Anybody needs the liberation from a conditional human existence; the only difference is that yogi seeks for freedom consciously while ordinary person does the same intuitively. But at this point nobody can get away clear with a help of relaxation, though it let to obtain a glimmering of detachment from conditions. Relaxation at the end of practice is the crown of all practice, and Yoga fulfills for the sake of the end.

If you continue to live among human beings, then you should be aware about correct beginning and finishing of the periodical daily Yoga practice. At the start you need to prepare your body and energy for transformation, at the end you need to be ready for routine activity, and this opposite transition is also complicated. Almost in any Yoga style practice is finished with Shavasana ('corpse'), when you lay down on your back and spread sideward at acute angles all limbs. Sometimes you can change common Shavasana to the relaxation with raising your legs up on the wall. It is essential after a hard work with arching because you can press your back against the floor easier if you rise your legs up. You should do the same after a practice dedicated to standing asanas, when your legs quake with weakness, and temporarily it is desirable to decrease the stream of blood there. But this position is senseless and harmful after inverted asanas especially with advanced variations when the inversion is accompanied with a strong muscle tension.

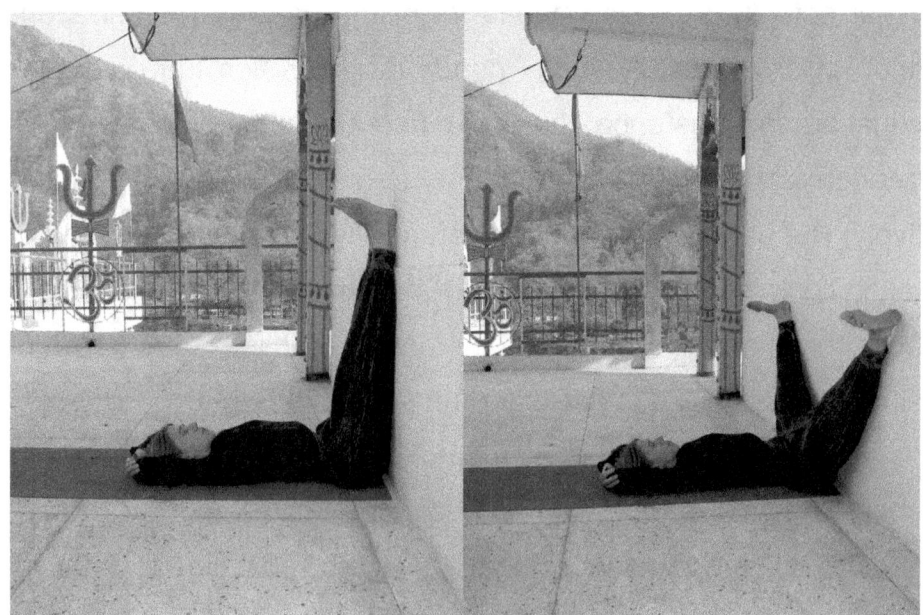

Photos 49-50

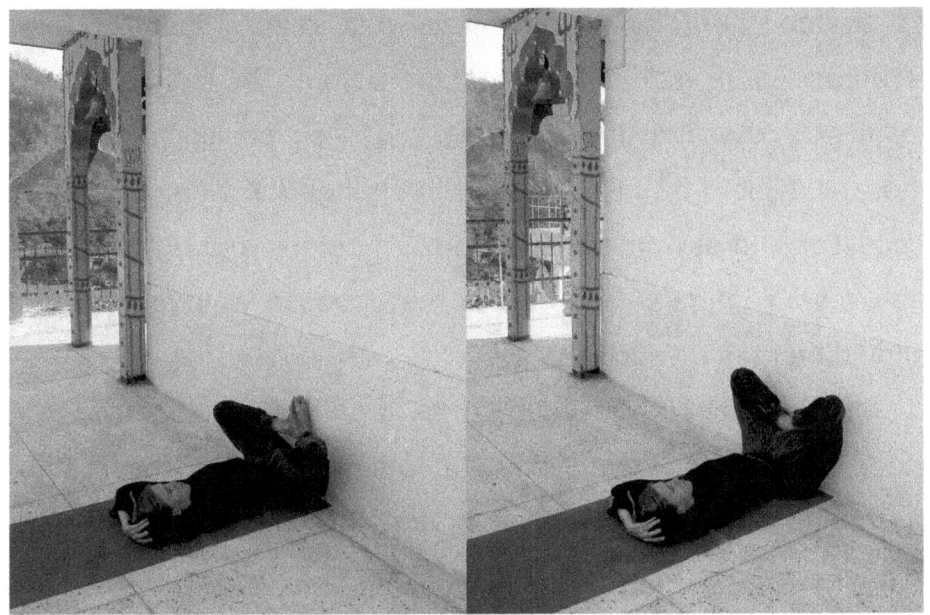

Photos 51-52

In order to use all benefits of relaxation with legs rose on the wall you can do the following sequence of postures, which is often use as a finishing in some Iyengar classes in Rishikesh. Take into consideration, that each position should be kept for some time, and don't change them one by one without any fixation otherwise the effect will be too insignificant. Lie down on your back moving your buttocks against the wall, then rise both straight legs up in vertical, join them closely and lean them equally to the surface of the wall (Photo 49). Pull your heels up and then completely relax the entire body. After some time separate erect legs aside as broad as possible at the current condition of your femoral arches (Photo 50). However don't try to stretch them at the moment, just relax. Then perform Bhadrasana as well as in handstand before (Photo 51), and after this Sukhasana that is simple cross-leg position 'sitting on the wall' (Photo 52). Don't forget to change the side, as always necessarily in asymmetrical asanas. If before your right leg was above your left leg, then now in the opposite way your left leg should be above your right leg.

Eventually bring your knees together, turn to the right side, wait a bit while your body becomes normal, and come up. According to another version of the finishing movement you should bend your legs, pull your thighs to your chest, rise your head to the knees and afterwards turn to the right side and so on. Anyway the position on the right side is very important and you must keep it sufficiently. On the one hand this posture helps to come back from the inner balanced state to the outer unbalanced world. On the other hand this posture helps to keep equilibrium grateful to the input of Ida-channel that is the lunar energy flow of appeasement.

Variations with Hinged Ropes

After the relaxation let us come back to the practice and include auxiliary facilities in it. Specific group of asanas is composed from variations with ropes fixed with one free end on the wall either above the head or at a waistline's level. Generally they are useful for better alignment, prolonged relaxation in inverted positions and deepening of arching and bending. Practically you can perform all the above-discussed types of asanas with a help of ropes, but here we confine ourselves to basic principles only. Still a rope on the wall is essentially different from the wall as such because a rope is artificial accessory, which is not seen in every house but you need to apply special efforts for its fixation. Moreover the workout with ropes is accidental operation in high degree, and you should practice it in a specially fitted hall under guidance of instructor. But this book is dedicated to homework. Nevertheless it is a good idea to bring away an overall impression about this approach to practice.

Usually in Yoga-hall there are two lines of hooks build into the wall for hanging ropes. One line is located at a waist's level, and another line is located above a head at a straight arms' high. The rope is never single but it always forms a large ply, which is useful as such otherwise you can keep both free ends in hands ignoring their connection. When you use a ply, it makes sense to put something like a folded blanket that the rope would not rip into your flesh. Sometimes you need to join ropes hanging from two nearby hooks, that the ply would be broad and not converging. Often you can see two plies hanging down from the same hook. This is very convenient if you need to keep a rope in two hands. In the case of the only rope your hands are necessarily one above another one, but then your posture becomes asymmetrical. But all that is joint moments of arrangement. Now let us talk why ropes are useful and what is possible to do with their support.

Rope for Grasp and Fixation

You can push the wall or lean against the wall, but you never could pull the wall closer since you are not able to catch a hold of the wall. True plane surface is main quality and unconditional benefit of the wall however sometimes it is not too convenient. Hinged ropes add dynamism for interaction with the wall keeping its stability. In other words your become more active in this interaction moving vertical line at your own will though you still continue to coordinate your movement with control surface. Subsequently we will talk about a special work with ropes in free space without any wall, but this is already an art but not the simple technique.

Additional Alignment in Standing Postures

Holding the rope you can align your body much easier in the postures, where the mastering depends on personal proportions namely the correlation of arms' and legs' length which are always unequal. Refresh your memory about form of asanas where it was required to put one leg on the wall holding its foot with the hand. The whole body became slightly warped since a leg is longer than an arm. But it is possible to escape this effect holding the rope because in that case you can find a proper distance between your hand and the wall. Both standing and sitting asanas require ropes fixed at the level above your head. Of course in the first case you will use ropes of higher line, while in the second case you will use ropes of lower line.

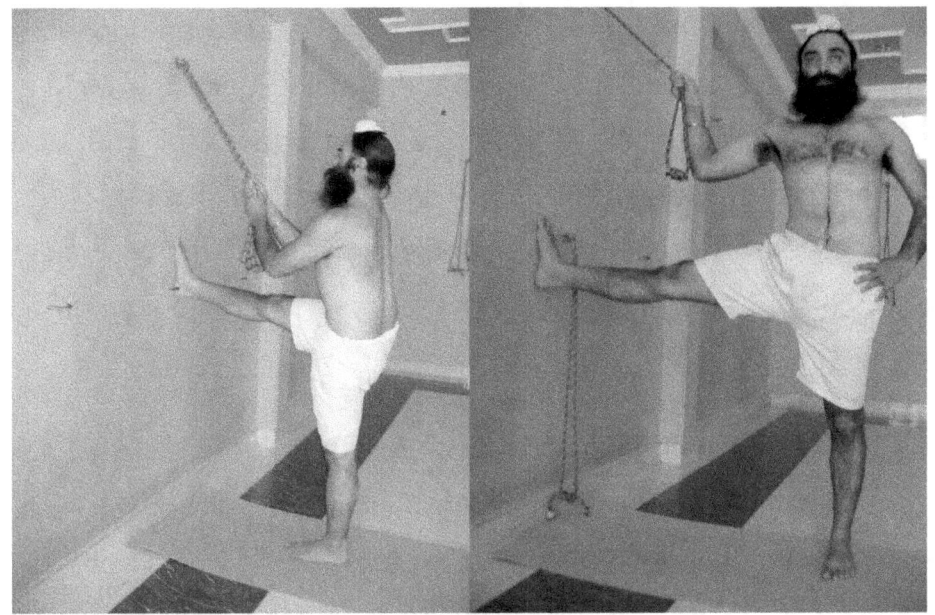

Photos 53-54

Let us come back to the very elements of practice that is alignment of the hips in standing asanas creating the right angle between leg and corpus. If you are holding the rope then you can keep the vertical position of your body as well pulling corpus closer to the wall and removing it back for correction. So, stand with your face against the wall, catch the rope, and put one leg on the wall at the right angle (Photo 53). Most probably you will find out that a position of your body is far from the ideal one that means your hips are not in line. In that case pull your corpus hitching the rope and simultaneously bending upper leg, then workout the correct position of your hips, and slowly straighten your leg without disturbing your hips. Repeat the same on the opposite side; after that workout a similar bending and unbending in stand with your side against the wall (Photo 54). Making variations you should be aware that your upper foot would be closely pressed against the wall independently on the movement of legs and corpus. The whole body is faultlessly straight and the axis is reclining totally like the inverted pendulum going back and forth.

Additional Alignment in Sitting Postures

Now let us do the same but sitting in front of the wall, therefore you should perform not reclining of the whole body but bending of its corpus only. You have to remember that your back must be straight in the process of bending. However it is a very difficult task, if you pull your corpus to legs holding your feet or toes. In that case your back hogs naturally, and maybe your spine's muscles are not strong enough that you could resist such an undesirable event. But situation becomes the completely different one if you pull your body snapping at a rope. Needless to say this is useful not for ultimate 'folding in twine' but for beginning mastering of bend, when even mitre angle is difficult. Holding the rope and pulling the body you achieve not too much inclination, but you keep a perfectly straight back and the stretched spine. It is much more essential than to touch your knees with your forehead. Additionally you are able to control the position of your hips stretching your legs and pressing both feet against the wall with thrusting off intention.

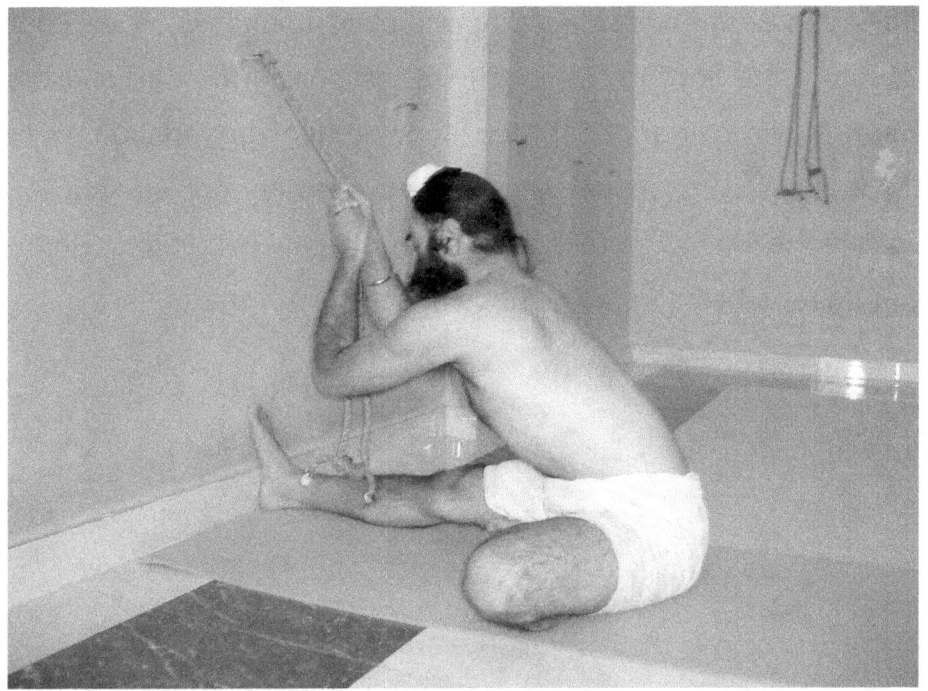

Photo 55

Also there is an additional advantage for the mastering of different variations of Janu Shirshasana that is the bending to one straight leg while another leg is bent by some means. Standard variations are Ardha Padmasana ('half-lotus') or Ardha Virasana ('half-hero', look the description of full Virasana). The simplest variation is the following: one leg is stretched forward while another leg is bent and put down aside with its knee on the floor and the foot is pressing the inner part of the first leg close to perineum (Photo 55). Astanga Vinyasa Yoga teachers add extreme variations with footstep like turning toes down and heel up or even toes back and heel forward. It is easy to get 'half-lotus' after performing the simplest variation: move your foot from the floor to the thigh, slightly pulling the calf and the knee closer to the straight leg. Independent of variations with the bent leg you should keep the thrust with your straight leg against the wall to correct the right angle between thighs. Snapping at rope helps for continuous reclining with straight spine.

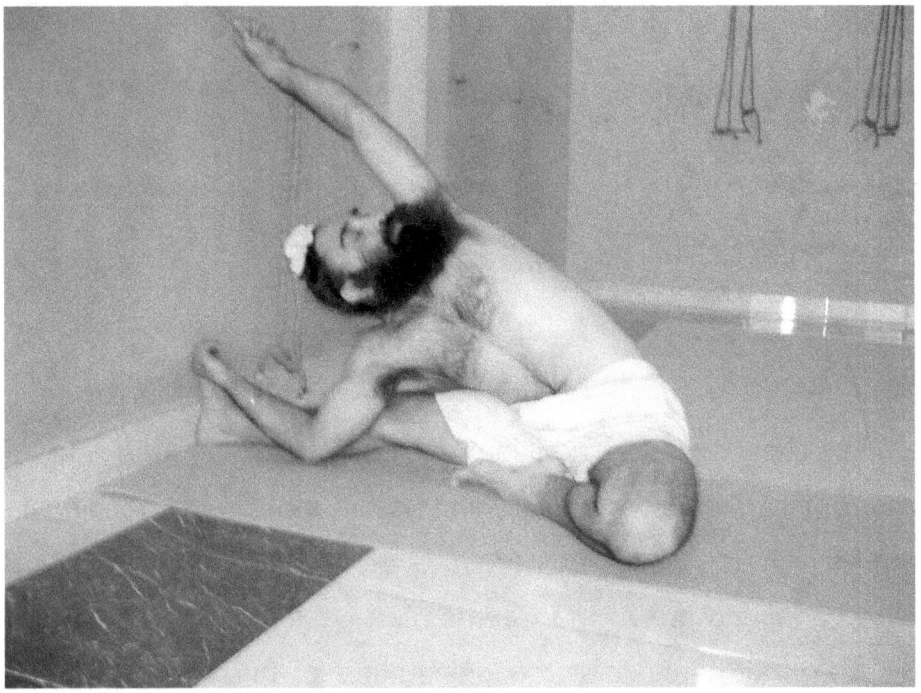

Photo 56

The bending makes sense only in the case if your hips are really aligned. For preparing you can lie down without changing the position of both legs and make the following exercise. Bend one leg, take another rope, fix ply on the foot, stretch the leg again, and pull it with the rope. You need find out equal positions of hips and perfectly the right angle between upper leg and corpus. As you did before you can slightly bend upper leg, correct your hips, and straight the leg again. If your hips disobey and remain warped, then you can ask someone to pull the upper thigh downwards using one more rope's ply. First of all your assistant puts the broad ply around your thigh close to the corpus. Then he puts his own leg inside of the ply at the same level above the floor, and goes back step by step till tension becomes extreme. Both participants should control the process because you feel the inner coordination of your limbs while the helper observes the exterior form sideways.

Eventually staying in the same position namely sitting in front of the wall and performing Janu Shirshasana you can add twisting (Photo 56). As discussed the above the stretching and straightening of spine column is the main preliminary condition for the mastering of twisting. That is why you should continue aligning your body pulling the rope with one hand, and at the same time you should put another hand on straight leg in order to produce an effort for body's twisting. At that you should try to move the knee of the bent leg as back as possible opening hips and creating some space for twisting in lumbar part of the spinal cord. Theoretically it must be done in one movement all over: spine's rotation proceeds because of removing leg, and the deeper spine twisting the wider hips opening, but anyway the knee should touch the floor all the time. If you succeed to put your elbow on the floor from the inner side of straight leg, then you can belay a palm under your head in order to force the twisting in thoracic part of the spinal cord. Also you can ask someone to promote the turning of your chest and hips using another rope for this purpose.

This is not the only sitting asana with twisting, and you can find out different variations with a rope in other postures. But always remember that performing all these movements you should continue to hold the rope with your upper hand and pull your body towards the wall. Thus you will master twisting exactly along the axis, but it is the most essential!

Rope for Rise and Extension

There is another wall's disadvantage also. The only possibility for spine's extension is limited to a partial carry of your upper body's weight. Certainly you can supply wall's defect merely if you snap at a rope higher or even at the hook itself and hang on the fixed point bending your legs. If you are positioned with your face against the wall then you should just bend your legs in the knees' joints. But it is not convenient if you are hanging with your back against the wall. In that case you should cross your legs and pull them up. Anyway you will achieve the effect of spine's stretching though without any use for a support of the wall. This is the basic concept, but adding variations with ropes fixed in the wall you can get spine's stretching in many different postures.

Obviously we find out the important dissimilarity from the previous working method with rope. Before you pulled your body using a manual effort but now the body is stretching under its own weight. Of course, such an extension is stronger but it can be controlled in a less degree. Nevertheless you still have area of support for limbs therefore there is some possibility for the correction. There's still a long haul ahead till unsupported swinging, and we are going to observe it separately. Also there is a tendency to arching or bending in all similar positions, however they are not suitable for deepening of round forms, and we'll talk about a mastering of the arch later. At present the only thing namely an ultimate extension of spine column by gravity is essential in different asanas.

Extension with Tendency to Bending

A low-fixed rope is convenient for spine stretching in bending with your back to the wall. The simplest one is the bending in 'down facing dog', where you need just put the rope's ply around your thighs close to your hips and bend forward (Photo 57). Find such a body's position that your feet would be fixed on the floor, your legs would pull the rope forward, and your entire corpus proceed to stretch forth. Thus your body hangs loose from the rope straining down and ahead until your palms will touch the floor as far from the wall as possible. Of course first you may bend and put your palms on the floor at any place and then you should gradually move your hands alone the floor on outreach. Do whatever you like but try to keep the final position as long as possible. In the common "dog" you form a 'triangle' with your tail bone as top grateful to muscular efforts. But here 'triangle' is constructed by itself because of relaxation and extension since top is strictly fixed by rope's ply.

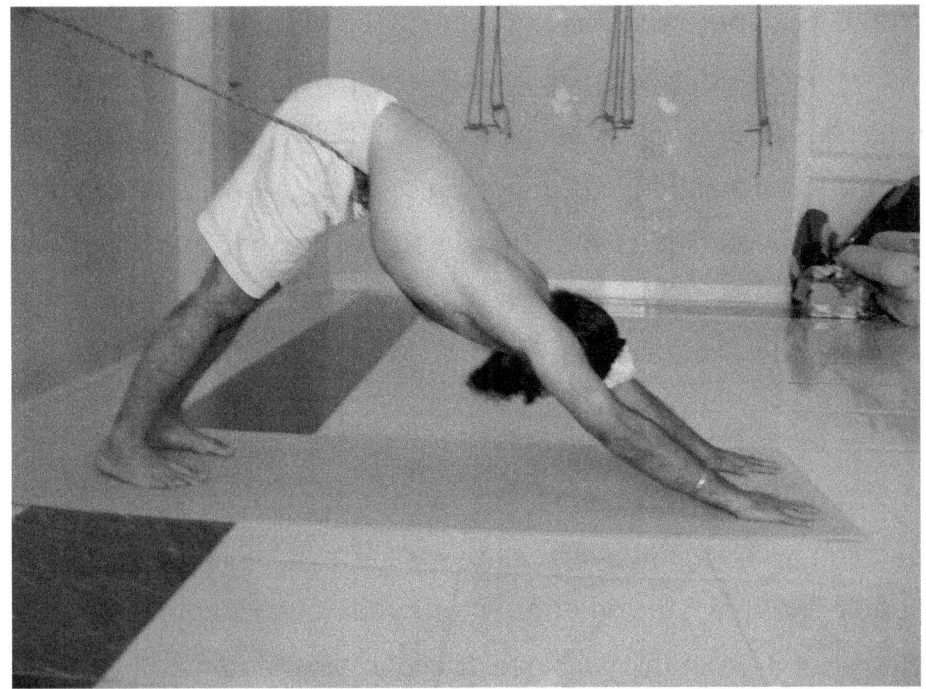

Photo 57

At this point we are getting on theme of forward bending with a straight back. It is good if a length of the rope's ply allows pressing your feet against the wall. Then you can immediately increase the effect and proceed to inclined variation of Padangushtasana. Bend more below and move you palms on your ankles pulling the entire corpus to your legs. Or move your palms alone the floor step by step reaching your feet. Remember that your back should be erect, and the bending is located mostly in hips' joints. Namely such a rope's position will give you an insight into the effect of folding in twain by the best way. If you have an assistant, then ask him to stand with his back against your back, slightly crouch, and press back to back. Thus you will be able to bend much deeper under his body's weight. Besides he can perform the same Padangushtasana too, using your back as 'wall'. Go back to the above subject with detailed description of forward bending with one's back against the wall.

There is another variation for deepening of the same 'down facing dog' posture. You can stand your feet on the wall with your toes against the floor or little bit above. It is important in the very beginning when anyway you are not able to put your heels on the floor. Moreover you may use different methods of fixing a rope around your body. First, you can make two plies and put them crosswise around opposite thighs. Second, you can put the middle part of the rope on the small of your back, turn both free ends around thighs inside, and pull them together backwards to the wall. The first is promoting of hips opening while the second is promoting of hips closing. The question is what you really need at the moment specifically according to the stage of practice. You can squeeze a wooden block by your thighs in the middle way between hips and knees. It will help you to control the work of your muscles. The effort to keep block is equal to the correct stretching of your legs in the pose, which let you to keep a proper form.

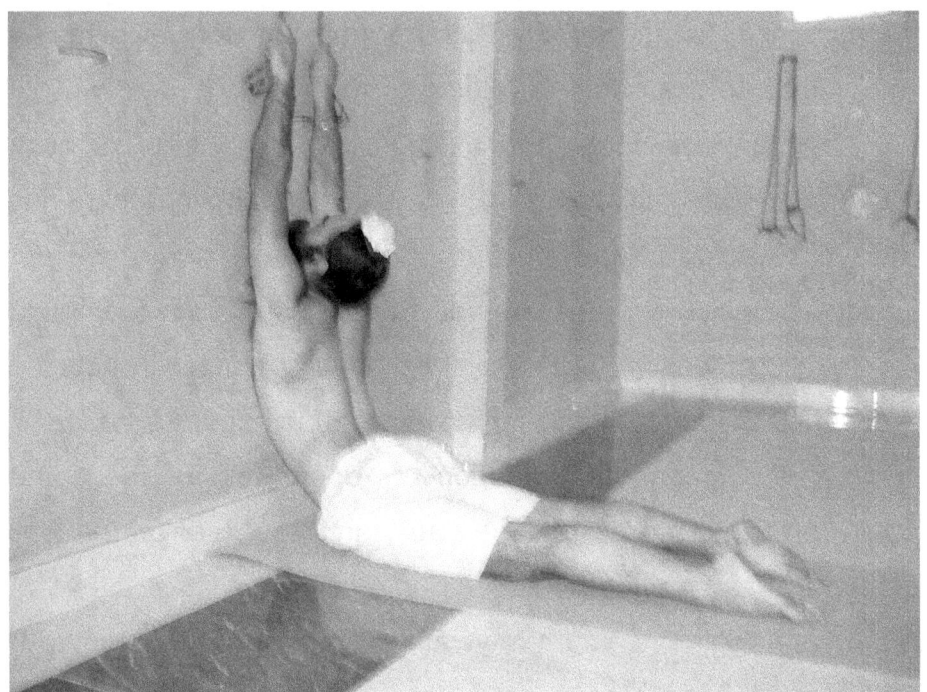

Photo 58

Extension with Tendency to Arch

Let us proceed from bending to compensatory action on the body. High-fixed rope is suitable for stretching with slightly arching. Firstly stand with your face to the wall in short distance and catch both free ends as high as possible. Then hang on all over until the rest with the forward body's surface against the wall without displacing feet and bending legs. Lastly start to slide down with your palms alone the rope in a smooth flowing manner moving your corpus us down us possible simultaneously pulling your legs off the wall. The limit of the movement is happening at the moment when your waist is located just the opposite right angle between the wall and the floor (Photo 58). It goes without saying that your body is inscribed in the corner through an arc, and there is more or less sizable gap between your stomach and the corner. At the beginning you can put a roller under your knees that not move too low.

It's better if you perform such a hanging in any sequence after Urdhva Mukha Shvanasana ('upward facing dog') but before Bhujangasana ('cobra'). This middle pose is different from both other asanas only by the arms' position. But you can discriminate both asanas according to their leg positions: in 'dog' you keep all body's weight on your toes while in 'cobra' you press your legs against the floor from toes up to a pubic bone. Obviously the hanging is similar to 'dog' at the start but eventually it transforms into 'cobra'. That is the reason why it is suitable in sequence namely between these two asanas. In the triad when you perform "upward facing dog" you should keep a check on the following details of the pose: press your toes against the floor, pull your spine upward, open your chest, and put your shoulders downward. Also the buttocks' tension is necessary for the fixation of a lumbar spine, that arching would not become too much. However you should make the tension by an external thigh without turning them inside. When you are hanging on ropes you can ask somebody to bear against your back in a down-forward direction. But previously you should learn to keep buttocks' tension otherwise the assistant will hurt your spinal column quite soon and easily.

After reaching the lowest limit at sliding alone the ropes you can proceed to deep Bhujangasana ('cobra'). Quit hold of the ropes since your entire body has already closely inscribed through an arc into the right corner between the wall and the floor, and rest for some time making the elbow lock above your head. Put massively your elbows and forehead on the wall to relax your whole body completely but don't proceed to the next movement prematurely. Then abut your hands against the wall at the proper level and gradually remove your upper body from the wall as far as possible. Be very careful and never do any movements asides because in that case the arching is even less than the right angle between your back and legs. At arching spinal bones are pulling together and any curving can lead to a cramp or trauma. Of course your feet should lie on insteps since in such an extreme position the additional uplift on toes would be felt as too sensible.

No matter where is your personal limit of flexibility you should be very attentive at the output from this posture. Even if you didn't perform a 'cobra' and continue hanging on the ropes then you must release the ropes to come back to the normal position. At the moment the pressure of your own weight can become unexpected overmuch. If you feel something like this then you must stay on arching pose none unwanted second. It is strongly not recommended that you would do what usually first come to mind namely turning aside. If the hall's floor is slippery enough then the best decision is the following. Push off the wall with your hands, move alone the floor all over, and lie down on your stomach in order to relax your spine totally. Otherwise you should pass your body's weight on your arms standing on the floor, bend your legs and sit on your heels. Finally low your stomach on your knees, put your forehead on the floor, relax in 'child' pose. After all performance some slight twisting in sitting position.

Rope for Deepening of Arch

Though 'cobra' belongs to real back banding, in the above case the rope served nothing but support for the preparatory stage. However the asana itself was performed after leaving the rope and pushing from the wall. Nevertheless you can start from another origin position and use the rope in special manner for deepening the arch, which is quite difficult without any support. We are not going to answer the question: 'Why to deepen the arch?' since the debate in Yoga literature on an issue continues until now. Obviously deep arching finds practical application in art and dance, but 'action-oriented' Yoga always transgresses into misinterpretation. In real practice the general submission is the flexibility of the spine as principle physics for development of energy structure based on the vertical axis Sushumna located directly inside of the spinal column.

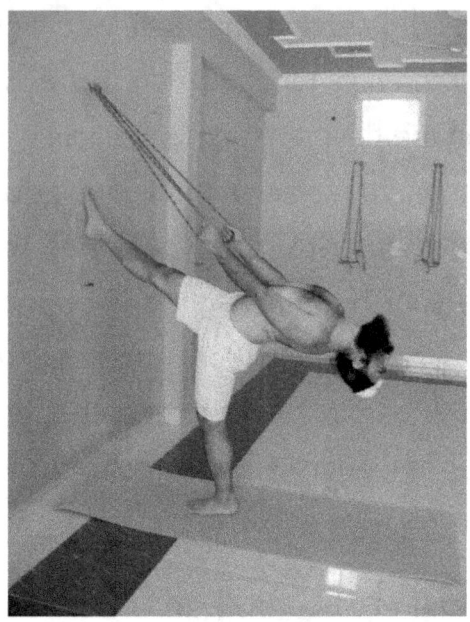

Photo 59

I believe that after all the above there is no need in any explanation for performing the arch in standing position when you press one leg against the wall, snap at a rope and decline your corpus backward (Photo 59). You are able to check the alignment of your hips, the stretching of spine, the keeping your head in line with your body, and so on. However the next type of arch is more complicated since you should press your feet against the wall and hang with the small of your back on the rope's ply. (Photo 60). As a preliminary you may put your heels on the floor in the only case if you have enough long rope. Also you may put a blanket under the rope to prevent your flesh from a rip. Keep a check on the correct rope's location, namely the ply should be not on the waist but on the upper hips, otherwise you will get not arch but a break of the spine. At the same time you must not take a risk that the ply would slip down otherwise you will pitch on your head. Don't forget to stretch your arms forward achieving even arch in thoracic spine as well to push with your feet from the wall. In other words, you should not just release your body and hang loose, but every part of the body fulfills the definite operation. The plain truth is that the asana is not suitable for relaxation.

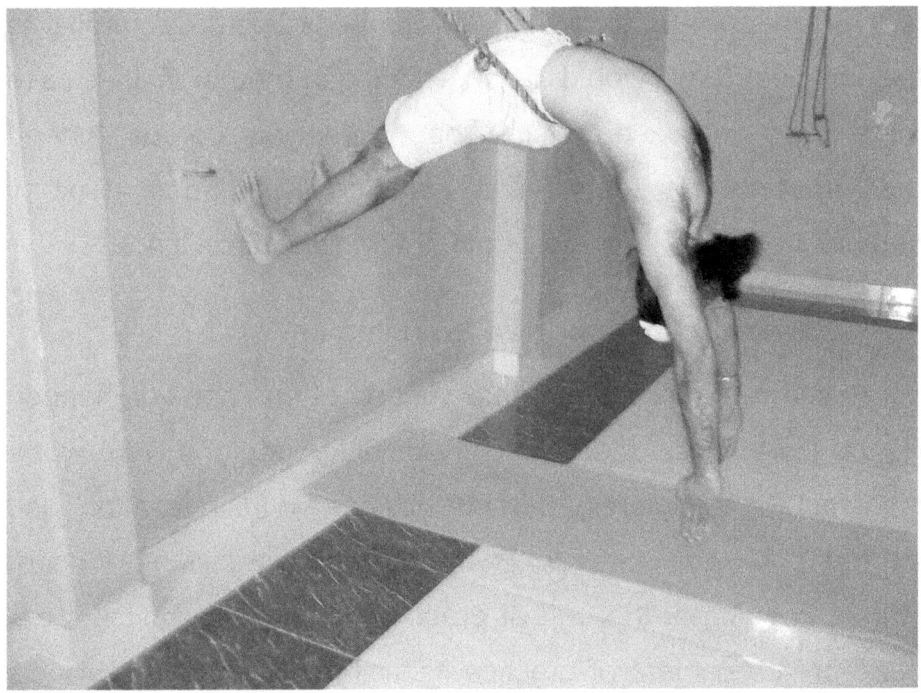

Photo 60

Herein we add the posture for compensation of extreme arching with similar extreme bending. Usually even under the instructor's guidance this pose is performed with a help of two-three people standing asides and behind the practitioner. That is why we give this description only for the completeness of this sequence but not as practical recommendations for individual mastering. This is inverted Pashchimottanasana (folding of body in twine) however not on the floor but in space. The only areas of support are the rope's ply under your back and feet pressing against the wall while the entire legs are pulled from the above to the front corpus. As a result whole body is strictly parallel to the floor as if you would lie on your back though in that case there is nothing except of the rope under your corpus. Indeed the output into this position is too much difficult and we don't try to describe it here that you would not try to perform it solo.

Rope for Unsupported Hovering

Almost in all cases with a support of the rope you hanged on the ply in some measure, but mostly your limbs were working. Now we are interested in possibilities for full relaxation, and we found two options only. Both positions are suitable for prolonged keeping at the end of practice though the choice is depend on the content of practice itself. In both cases the rope's ply is embracing your body thus your can completely relax but your pose will not be changed and you can be sure that the ply will not be removed from the proper place. Even any support of the wall is not very important.

The first variation is good enough as compensation after arching; however it's better if you control the rope with your hands. It's desirable that you pass your arms round the rope which is stringed. (Photo 61). In order to relax after performing the arch with a ply on the small of your back you can use inverted Paschimottanasana also without leaving the ply. Straighten your trunk, put your feet on the floor, turn with your back to the wall, bend downward, interlock your elbows, bend your legs, and press your front calves against the wall. In this position there is no need to workout the proper bending since your stomach will squeeze up against your thighs naturally. As a result whole body is hanging and you are facing the wall. Your assistant can do the same like before, namely he pushes back to back, that you could move your shoulders and chest close to the wall. Thus you perform well-known 'child' pose not on the floor but on the wall.

The second variation is useful as a substitution of headstand (Photo 62), which is usually completes the active practice just before finishing with Shavasana. It is good for people with spine's problems especially in the cervical part. They get the effect of the inversion in the full measure, at the same time there is no any pressure on the back. Quite opposite, they get intensive stretching which is always healing for the spine column. Merely put your feet together and knees aside that the rope could press your thighs against the wall. In this position the hanging is more safely than in the first case, however you can arch your back a little bit that the ply would be located in slight deepening. Principally there is the only recommendation: just relax your whole body.

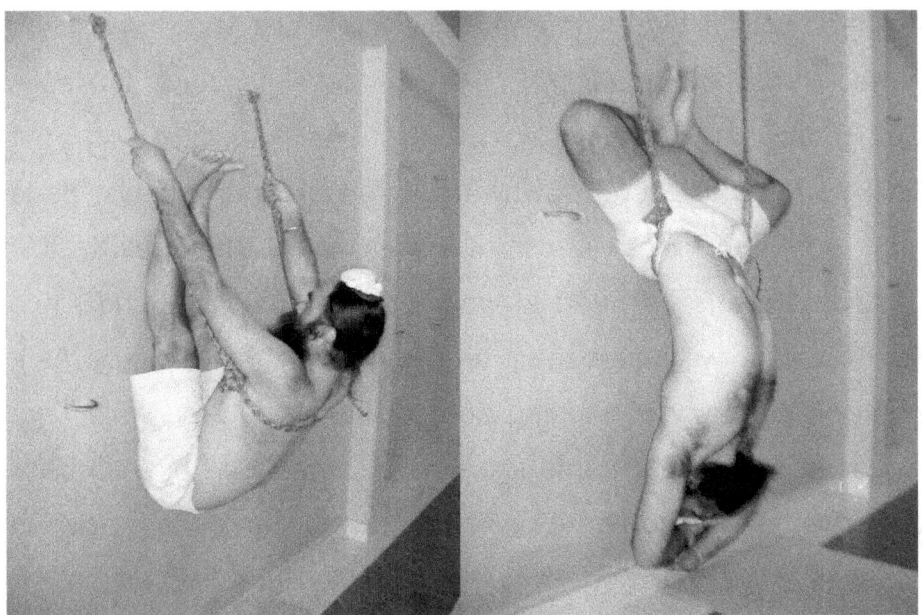

Photos 61-62

Part III.
Advance: in 'Free Flow'

Wall is metaphorical 'dead end', and flow is metaphorical 'path'. However the world is not a black-and-white movie, and there are many intermediate forms of existence between such extremities as presence of the wall and absence of the wall. In Russian Yoga the 'free flow' is a modern term with ambiguous and polemic content, and we apply it as a designation for an intermediate stage. In our context the path is vertical; therefore 'free flow' supposes just a kind of liberty in the interaction with the wall. Otherwise you can accept it as considerably expanded conception of the wall itself, but such understanding has almost the equivalent action's potential. So, let us answer the question which abilities are appearing when the wall (existing in consciousness and reality) becomes more shaky and mobile?

The very evident achievement is the discovering of the inner deepening of the space, which is limited by the wall. Then you don't lean against the wall turning a blind eye to the whole world but you put the wall at the proper place. You take into account the existing of emptiness before the wall and find a possibility for using this space. You can combine asanas against the wall with asanas in the distance, you feel free coming close to the wall and going away from the wall. Moreover hinged ropes can take the place of the wall generally in the sense of vertical, and thus you proceed to the style Mallakhamb. Finally, you notice that wall's surface is not necessarily even. So, you can pass to practice with rocks and other relief objects, where vertical and horizontal are transgressing into each other naturally.

Access to Wall - Recess from Wall

After observing asanas according to the types of 'body pressure on the wall' we can conclude that the wall is a useful support for all standard asanas' types such as bends, arches, twists, inverted and balancing poses. The entire spectrum testifies that we can include practical work with the wall not only into the mastering of separate asanas but also into the constructing of sequences. It is inevitable, and we could not ignore the order of asanas even performing them separately. The same concerns the wall as 'corrector' or 'helper' for Yoga-teacher. You saw the constant appearance of variations where it was required to enter the information about making combinations. Thus we got short sets of asanas, and the same posture was alternatively performed either next to the wall or inside of free area, either with exterior assistance or on your own authority.

Learning combinations from two-three asanas and using the whole arsenal of wall-working techniques, you can proceed to create two-hour sequences. However herein we are not required to give different asanas' sets, it's enough to emphasize well-known wall-mastering aspects and put them into a distinct shape for the realization. That is why we just shortly recall and summarize the elements of asanas' combination and partner's work rambling among descriptions of separate asanas. There are three parameters only for the selection of constructive principles how to workout asanas' nets. In powers of complicated situation one may range them into the following order:

- independent performing of one and the same asana against the wall and in free space;
- alternation of secondary form with instructor's help and main form against the wall;
- alternation of similar asanas against the wall and in free space.

The wall as a function of correction can serve on the substitution of instructor, and at solo practice it is reasonable to perform the same asana alternatively against the wall and in the middle of the room. This principle is suitable for the mastering almost all asanas. The supporting wall's role is the most obvious when you need to align your whole body in the vertical plane, for example, performing 'triangles' where usually insufficient hips opening cause all over curving. You can master 'triangle' variations with your back or face to the wall. In the first case asana is aligning mostly by muscular efforts; in the second case the alignment is achieved owing to weight's pressure of the body leaned against the wall. That means in the first case asana is working out in the stressed state while in the second case full relaxation is required and arising.

If you are Yoga teacher yourselves, or you learn Yoga in groups, or just you prefer to make your home practice with a partner then you find out the second parameter. That means you can alternate any secondary position mastering with the assistance of your teacher or partner and the main position against the wall. In the process we noted many standing asanas where the wall is useful for the correction by Yoga-teacher also. For instance, when a disciple is performing Utthita Hasta Padangushtasana then his instructor can easily help him to remove an upper leg aside if he is standing with his back against the wall. So, Yoga-teacher presses his shoulder with one hand and pushes his foot or knee with another one. The remarkable wall-variation was demonstrated for the correction of Pashchimottanasana. Namely, the instructor performed handstand on the back of his disciple with the wall's support for his feet. Thus he combined successfully his body weight's pressure on the back with a possibility for alignment of each part of the back by his hands. You see, instructor would not be able to feel the skin and muscles just walking on the back with his feet. At the same time if he would workout the back with his hands standing on the floor then the pressure would not be strong enough.

The third parameter let you prepare to reject the wall in the case if you are learning to alternate similar asanas mastering them both against the wall and in a free space. Thus constructing sequences you include the process of wall-working into your common practice on the floor. In the course of operation you restore possibilities for a spatial motion limited by the wall. Studding asanas' interaction with each other you need to come close to the wall and go away from the wall. In what connection asanas are arranged in such a manner, that their effects resonate and increase reciprocally. You can use in the capacity of correlative asanas particularly Adho Mukha Shvanasana ('down facing dog') and Vrikshasana (handstand); Virasana (sitting between your calves) and Ardha Matsyendrasana (twisting against the wall with one leg in Virasana) and so on. How such twins work principally? In the first instance you align the correct position of shoulders; in the latter instance you give your attention to hips opening; but in the both cases the asanas' alteration promotes the perfection of each posture specifically.

We consciously investigated only a static style of practice, and even sequences were studied as passages from a distinctively fixed severe asana to another one. However there are dynamic styles also, where your movement is more important while separated asanas act just as a designation at start and finish. We described just two moments of such an approach and can remind them. In dynamic practice the wall can serve for a thrust or a stop-end in so-called 'whirling' asanas. While performing an output from Chakrasana back to handstand you can change the level on the wall which is suitable for transferring feet from an extreme low position to an extreme high position. This movement is the opposite one to the mastering of an input from Tadasana to Chakrasana, since in that case the wall is a support for feet instead of hands, and you are going to perform a symmetrical motion in the space. The wall starts to serve for such complicated functions in Ashtanga Vinyasa Yoga at the mastering of advanced sequences. But any props are not standard for this style, and the wall-working is not classical method.

Mallakhamb on Rope or Column

Suppose you perform the perfect Yoga practice with a support of the wall. Generally if you get over the wall and not intend to leave the wall, then you discover two ways of the development. Nominally we could associate them with an opposition between artificial and natural developments. In the first case the vertical is presented by a column or a rope, like in Mallakhamb-Yoga where asanas are performed in "suspension", the performance itself relates rather to Yoga-sport and dedicated to keeping an ideal physical form. Really this style is almost unknown in Russia even from books, except of a short article in Yoga Magazine as well as some pages with a historical summary in the collected volume *'Dynamical Practice in Classical Yoga'* (Kiev, 1999). Until proceeding to the core of a subject let us overlook how this style is connected with Iyengar Yoga, because herein we use some 'external techniques' of this Yoga school though assigning them a specifically different meaning.

All props including a wall and ropes were entered into Yoga practice by Sri Krishnamacharya, the guru of B.K.S. Iyengar. However research workers found medieval texts which looks as the source of his tradition, and defiantly he could obtain corresponding details from those books. Among them there are some rear texts such as *'Malla Purana'* and *'Shritattva Nidhi'* dedicated to a training of fighters. Revealingly there is photography in a book by Sri Krishnamacharya himself where we can see two ropes hanging down from a ceiling. Therefore he really used ancient wrestler's methods in Yoga practice. Moreover the tradition itself was reborn in Mysore where Sri Krishnamacharya taught Yoga. In Maharashtra state the Mallakhamb style has survived till our times, and every year they hold competitions in movement alone the column. The origins of this wrestling art are trace back till the text *'Manasolhas'* dated at 1135 AC.

The chapter 10 of *'Malla Purana'* (XII-XIII AC) contains 16 classes of exercises which were popular at that time, including *stambhashrama* on a column. There are 4 types of support for these movements: on a thick oiled column embedded below the ground; a column in the similitude of a stick; a construction from two hanged columns; a long stick. The subsequent text *'Shritattva Nidhi'* contains many 'bird's' asanas performed on the rope but obviously originated from hanging wrestler's columns. Probably they were useful even for training of English soldiers stormed Indian forts. Until now you can listen to a legend how soldiers tied a rope to a lizard and cast it on a villein wall. When it clawed hold of the wall strongly, fighters climbed along the rope, and the fort was conquered. Maybe the storm of walls with ropes was the necessarily element of a battle training.

After some time the walls' storming became already non-topical but the rope training was proved to be essentially tenacious of life owing to its artistry. I was lucky to watch the performance of Edgar Ortize (Photo 63), the Iyengar Yoga instructor from Costa Rica. First I should notice neoclassical character of this demonstration since it was done far not on column or rope. A long bright-colored width was hanged down from the thick branch of a great tree at the level of the third floor in such a manner that both free ends hanged loose till the very ground.

From the farness it was non-comprehensible what is happening there. A man literally slipped along the width from top to bottom smoothly hovering in the air (Photo 63-a). The upper part of the width really became like two ropes under his weight, while both lower free ends trembled by indescribable iridescent waves from each his ingenious movements (Photos 64, a-b).

It would be just a quite good show however his movement was the ideal performing of advanced asanas. As you know, Iyengar style is glorious by asanas mastering, and in that case the mastery was kept faultless even upstairs. Later I got a possibility to estimate Edgar Ortize's perfection in handing of technical shades when I visited his class. There were already nothing vertiginous, but some material on the practice with a support of the wall was accepted namely from his teaching.

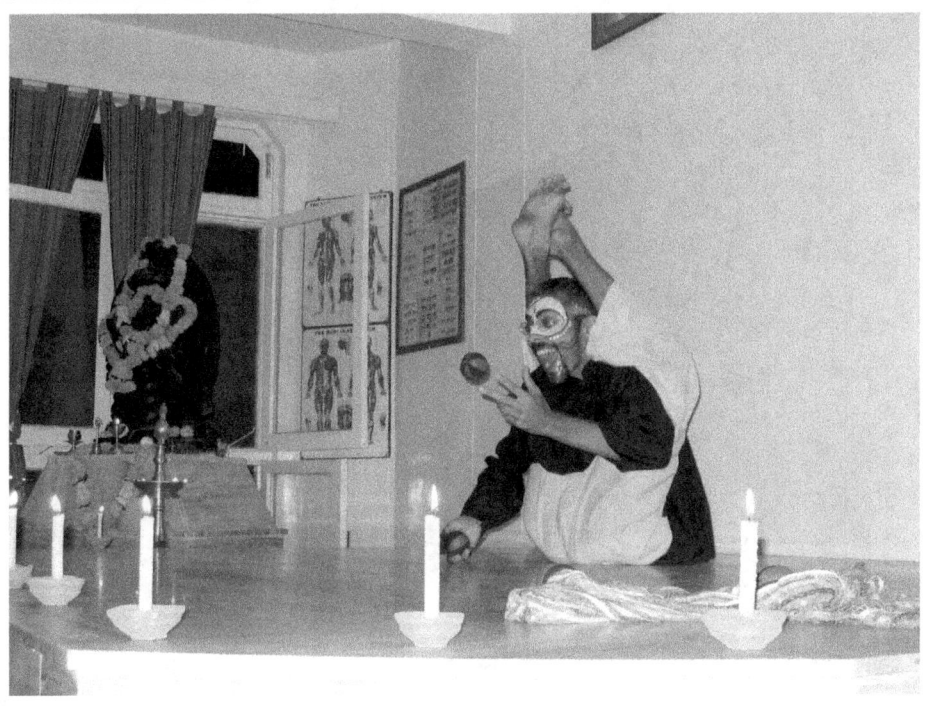

Photo 63

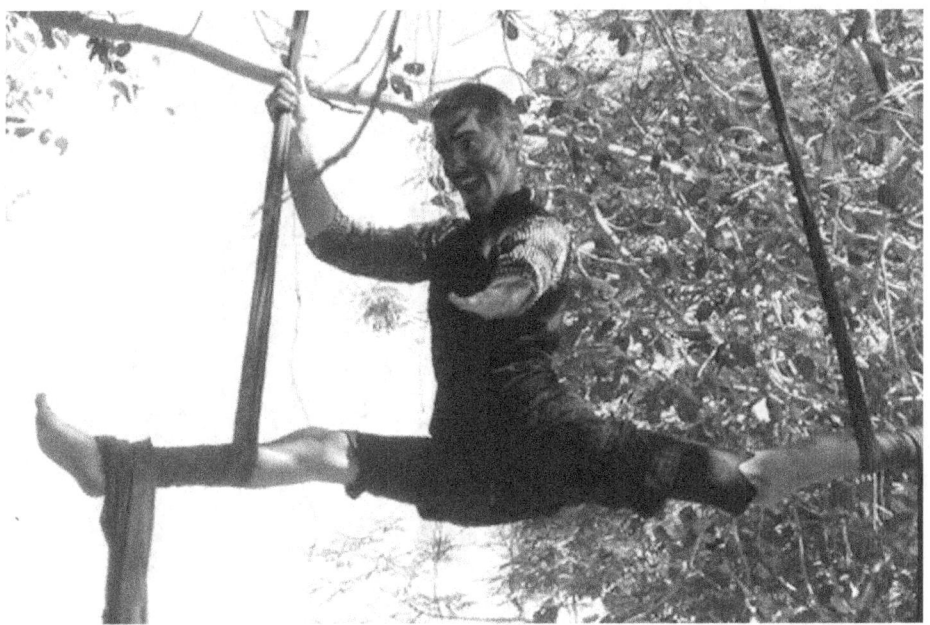

Photo 63(a)

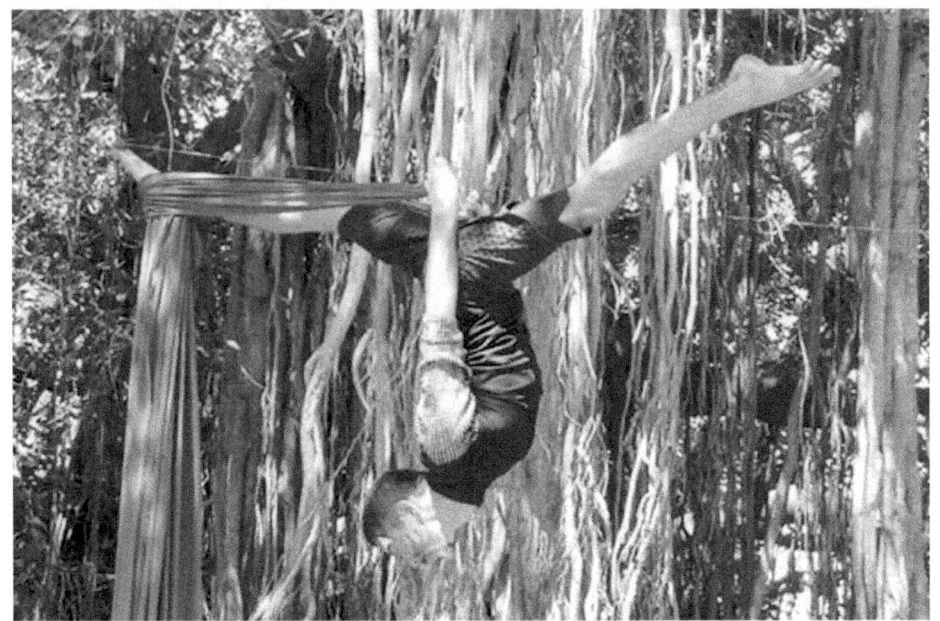

Photo 64

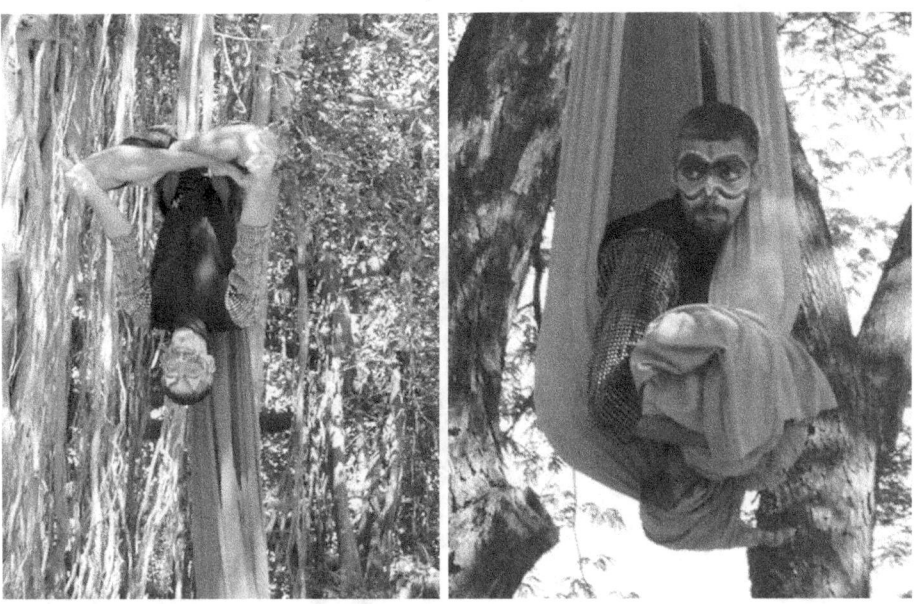

Photo 64 (a-b)

Thus, swarming against the wall seemed to be a mark of irresistible infirmity, however in point of fact it turned out to be directly associated with an admirable body-control in flight.

Especially the inverted and arching asanas outlook in the midst of everything, that sank into the mind voluntarily at the performance. Of course, inverted positions in hanged state were easily achieved by sheathing of widths around legs rather by coiling of legs around widths. Replacing the plies close to hips he was able to perform even a cross split at inverted body orientation. Such arches like 'cobra' were fulfilled in the same manner as on the floor. His body was sheathing all around at the hips level, the arms clambered a rope above his head. As a result the arch was amounted to the right angle between his back and legs, but sometimes it was reduced to the oblique angle. The 'tortoise' was used by the way of compensation, though it's difficult to master it even on the floor. This is extreme banding, when the corpus not only lie closely along the legs but proceed to the space between separated legs together with arms. Moreover the arms continue to move backward, turn around legs, and join behind the back while ankles are crossed behind the neck. Relatively speaking, it is preferable to catch a sight...

Even feeling the sincere admiration of such the mastery nevertheless I believe no matter to be big on the art or become an artist. Formal interest emasculates interpenetration of practice with awareness, but that is unreasonable price for the staginess. Therefore we are going to give you other non-classical ways except of return to classical Yoga itself. Yogic development must be mere conscious, intended to unity with Universe. Otherwise artistic investigations draw out chiselled borders between the body and corporality as such. Simply stated, even adjustment of both Yoga and dance can be not suspended over viewers, but incorporated into the natural land's configuration, integrated into variable surfaces of rocks and trees.

'Dance Improvisation' with Rocks

The alternative choice is the practical passage from the even wall to a land configuration, where you will never meet direct horizontal and vertical planes. Any native habitat always includes different inclined planes at high-angle or low-angle over and above with an uneven surface. The art of improvisation is necessarily for the practice in such conditions among rocks or trees. However it is kept within the frame of standard movements though it gives a chance to perfect them till subtlest details. It seems you develop your own structure, but at the same time you master your interaction with an ambient energetic space instantiated by indeterminism. Namely this path looks like the most reasonable one in a perspective of gradual including of entire Universe into the self-conscious process. After achievement of the final goal that is Samadhi (concentration) all complete objective variety will be grappled in block. Herein I result the summary of my observation of Asana practice by Michael Jekel (Germany) on rocks of ocean coast and banks of Ganges.

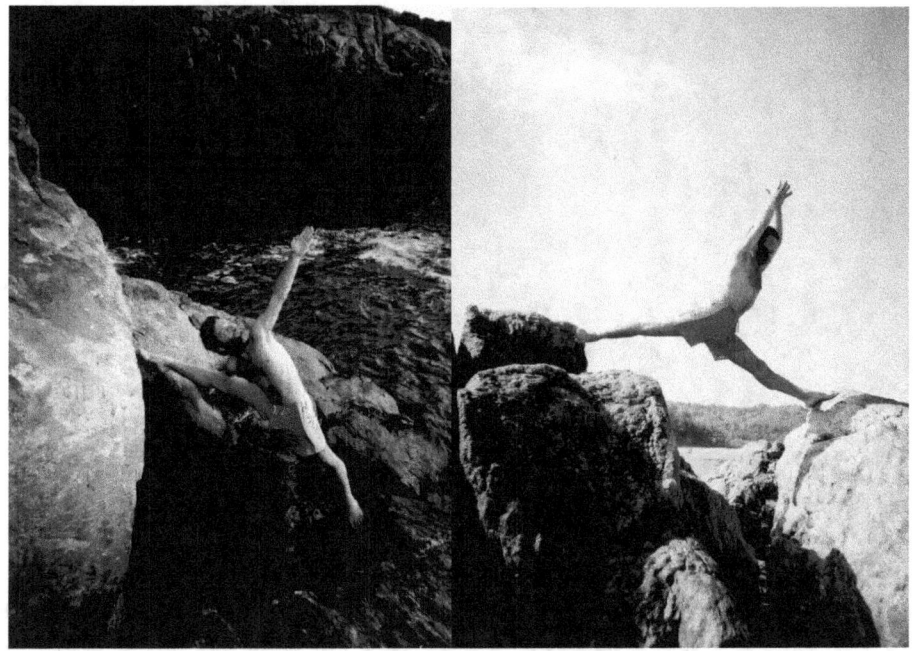

Photos 65-66

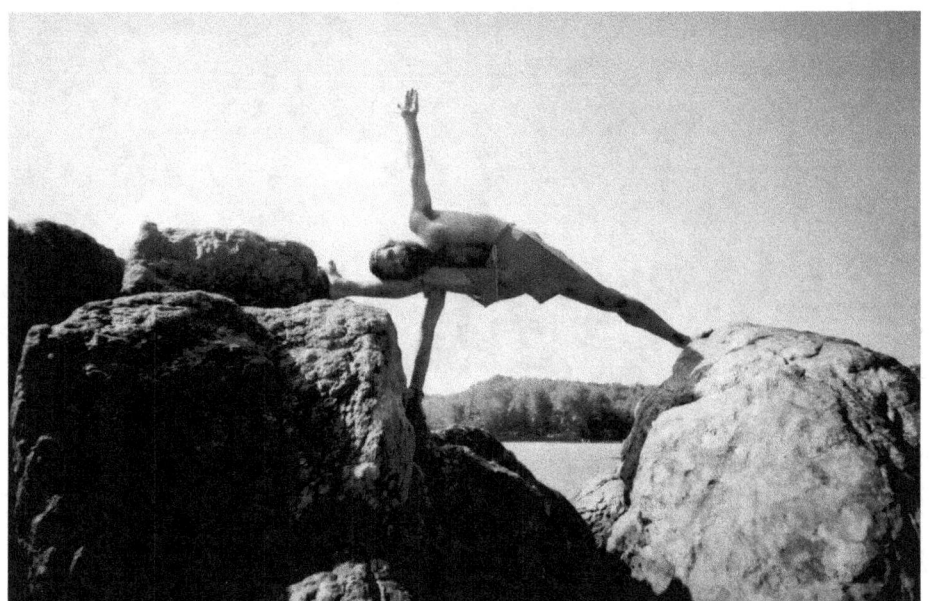

Photo 67

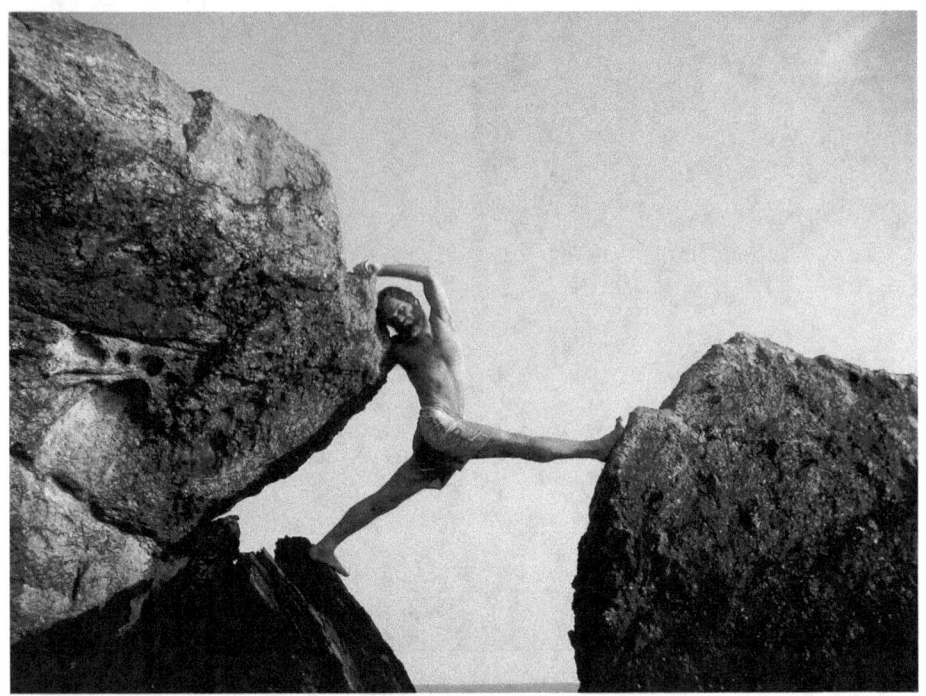

Photo 68

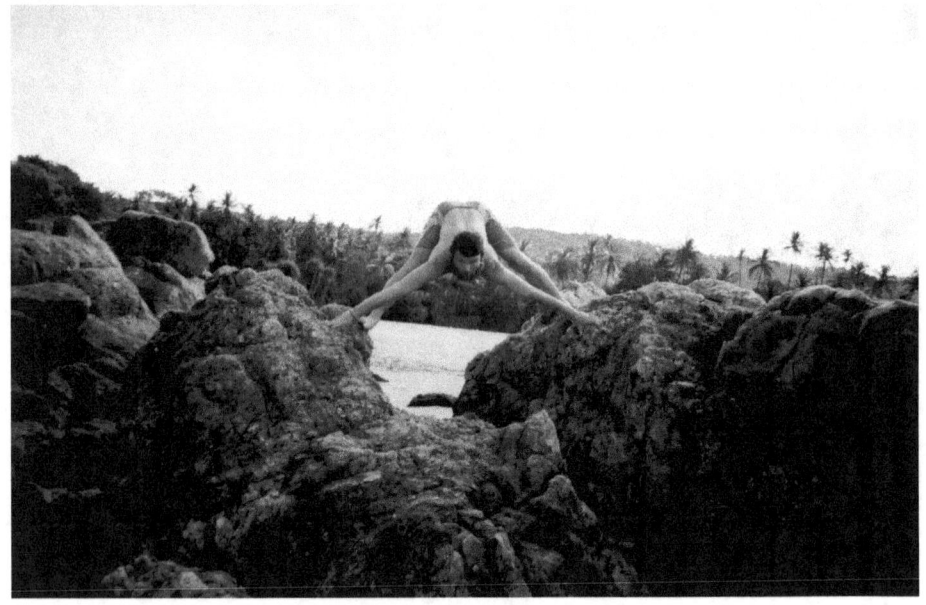

Photo 69

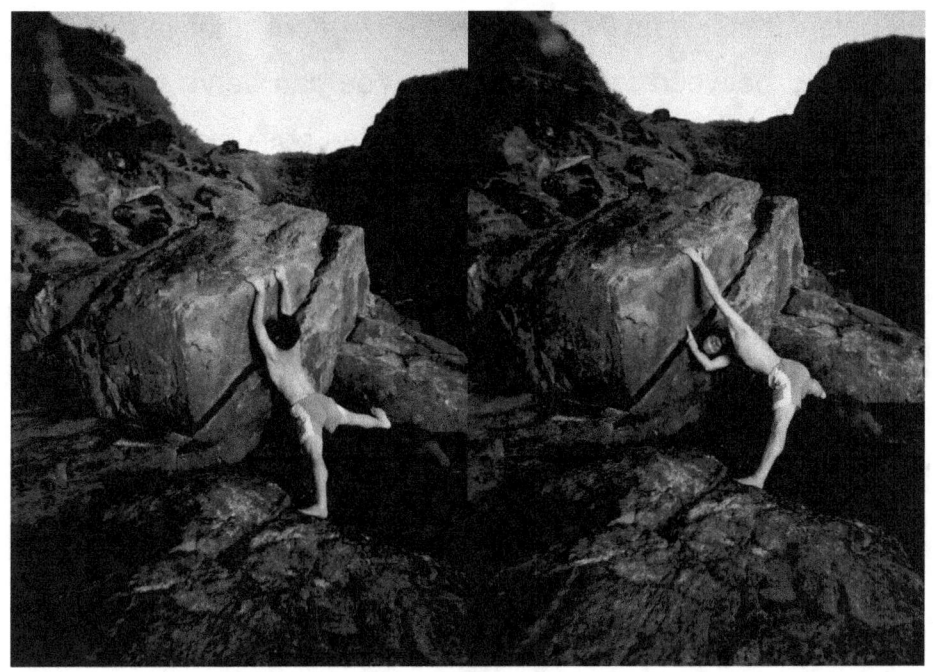

Photos 70-71

There is the simplest and the most obvious thing in rock's landscape, namely a sudden appearance of small gaps, which should be overstepped, though not always both edges are at the same level (Photo 65). Rocks can be at any distance from each other, while small sites which are convenient for footsteps can be higher or lower. In that case you get large amount of possibilities for mastering asanas with straddle up to forward and cross splits (Photos 66–67). Of course, a vertical extension of rocks on either side gives you a wide space for variations with your upper body, especially for twisting (Photo 68), but also bending and arching. Moreover, you will find out an absolutely unbeaten track, namely a space 'below floor' that is potholes downward between feet (Photo 69). You can bend and stretch in that direction refining asanas to inverted postures. In the case if a gap is bounded from three sides along the lines of 'semi-well', then you can put your feet on opposite edges and workout the middle wall turning with your back or face against its surface (Photos 70–71). Supplementary holding variations are approachable owing to all kinds of shelves in the absence of hanging ropes.

Fantastically incredible variations are created in gorge between two connivent walls, endlessly proceeding upward and downward. You can hang on such space only making 'flying shores' with your legs and arms placed on scarcely noticeable 'cling holds'. In that case it's enough to forget oneself and become inactive that crash down therefore concentration is not a problem (Photos 72–73). It is interesting to observe in such gorges the series on the base of Pashchimottanasana impacted between two rocks: feet are standing on one wall, hips are pressing against another wall, and corpus is settled on tensely straightened legs (Photo 74). It is noteworthy that some teachers recommend imagining of such pushing to opposite sides even for mastering this asana on the floor. But here it is quite inevitable and necessary for keeping configuration as well as holding body on two areas of support. Further in hold you can digest vicinity, making variations by means of free arms and corpus.

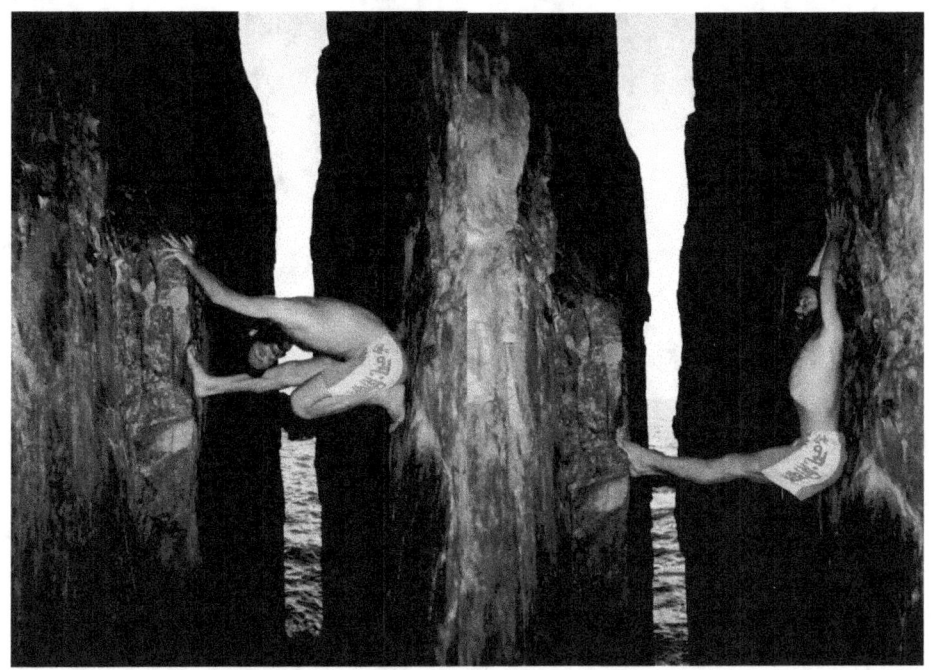

Photos 72-73

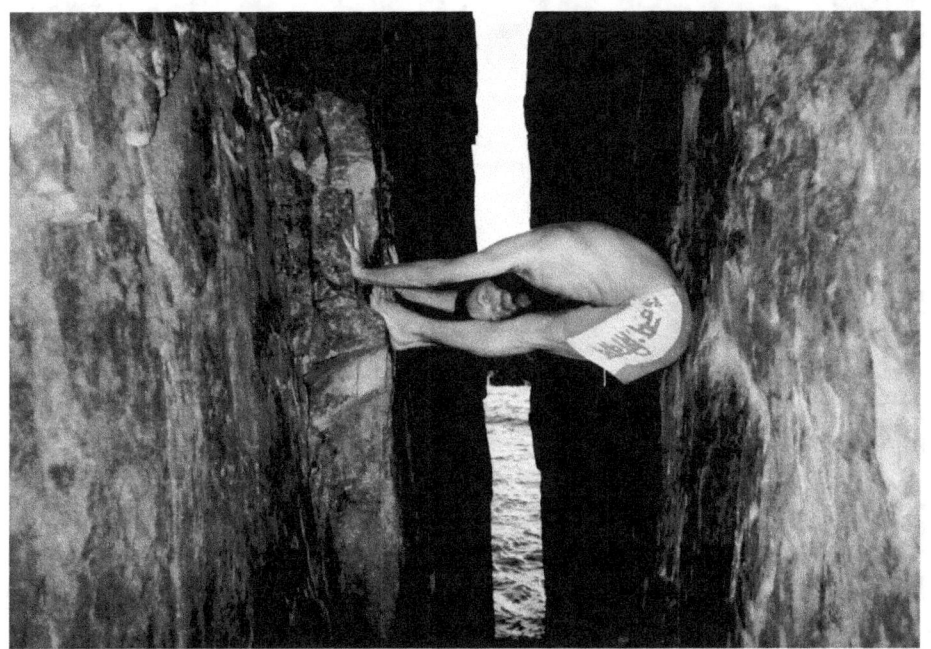

Photo 74

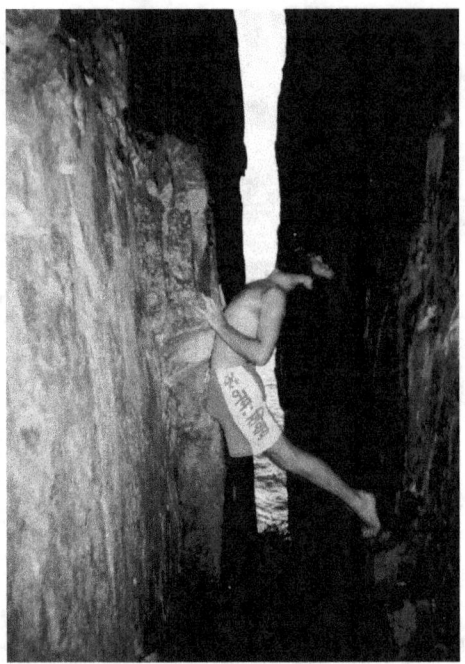

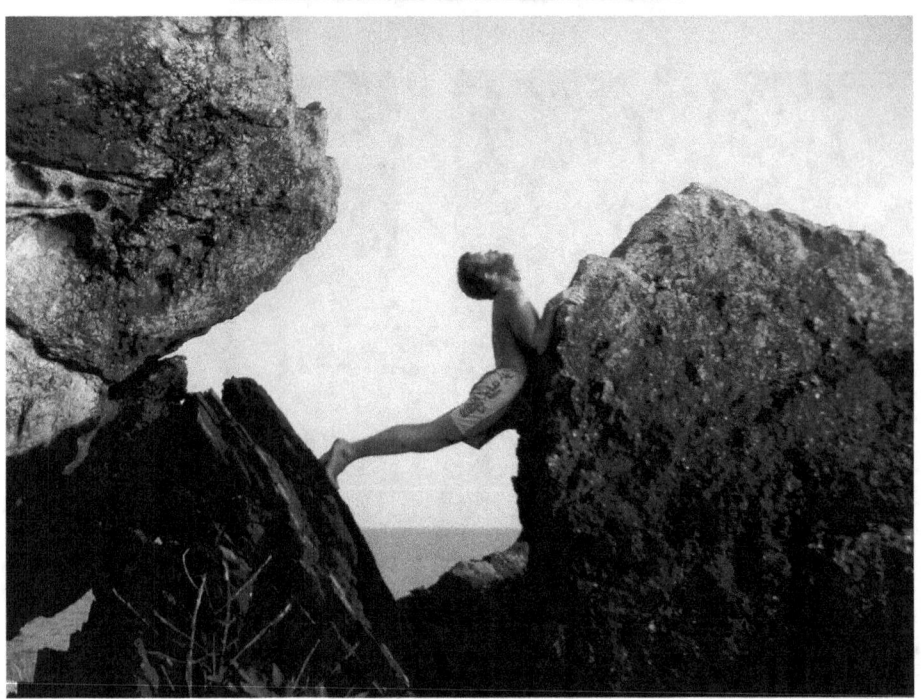

Photos 75-76

Arches look also variously on the rocks being at different distances. The simplest 'cobra' assumes an unusual view when it is performed almost in vertical (Photo 75). For this purpose you should put your feet on one wall of a gorge and press your front body against another wall. Then hands' thrust causes the reclining of the head backward till it touches the opposite wall strictly above feet. However if a distance between rocks is too long, you will get completely new asana, though from aside it seems exactly the same as 'cobra' on the floor (Photo 76). Usually your legs are lying on the floor and your corpus is arising above its surface, while now everything is going in the opposite way: your legs are stretched in the emptiness and your abdomen and low chest are pressed against a vertical rock. For sure, you will be required to find out other positions in space, except of described the above (vertical and horizontal).

You see, rocks are unpredictable; and you could find options even for whole classical sequences such as Surya Namaskara. Here we show the only two basic postures from it (Photo 77, a-b) though it consists from 12 poses. If you know this sequence you can imagine prolongation. Surya Namaskara serves as starting postures in Ashtanga Vinyasa Yoga also. Then you can do some standing asanas where you can use two different supports for feet (Photos 78-79) etc. There is now special benefit while you will get a new feeling of your body moving in space. So, you can choose some Asanas as you like according to any Hatha Yoga style.

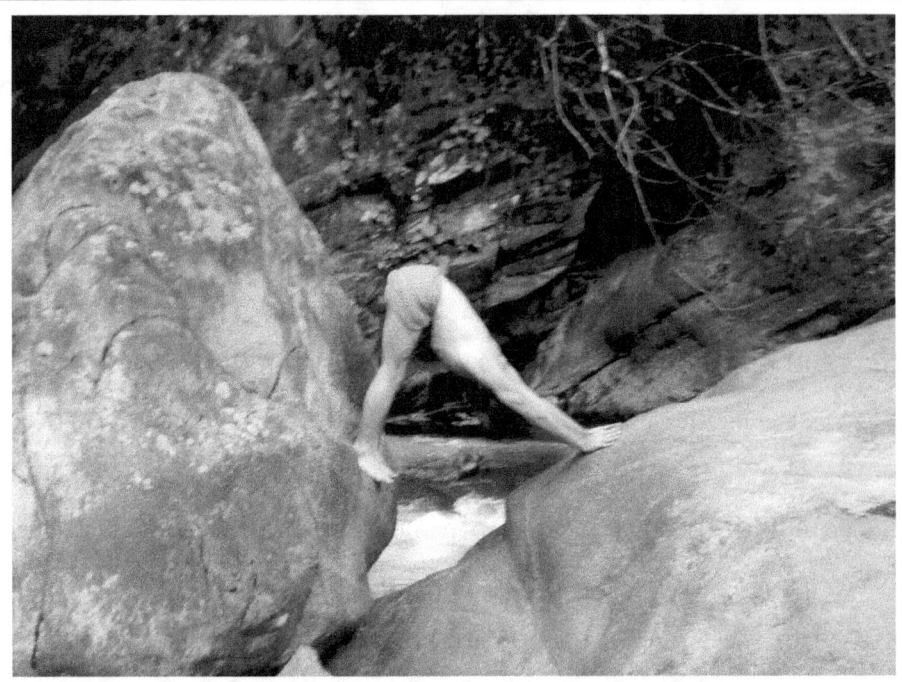

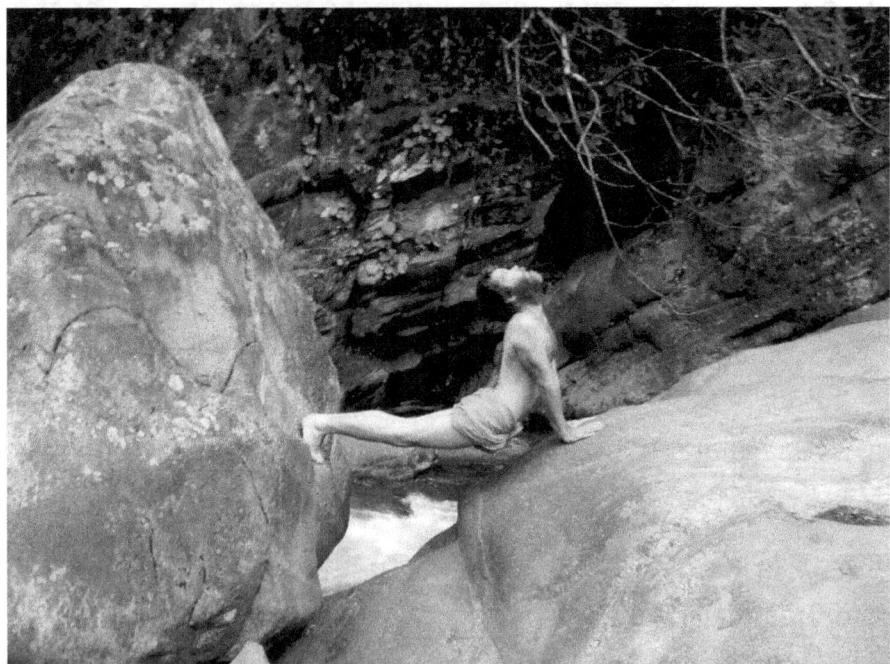

Photos 77 (a-b)

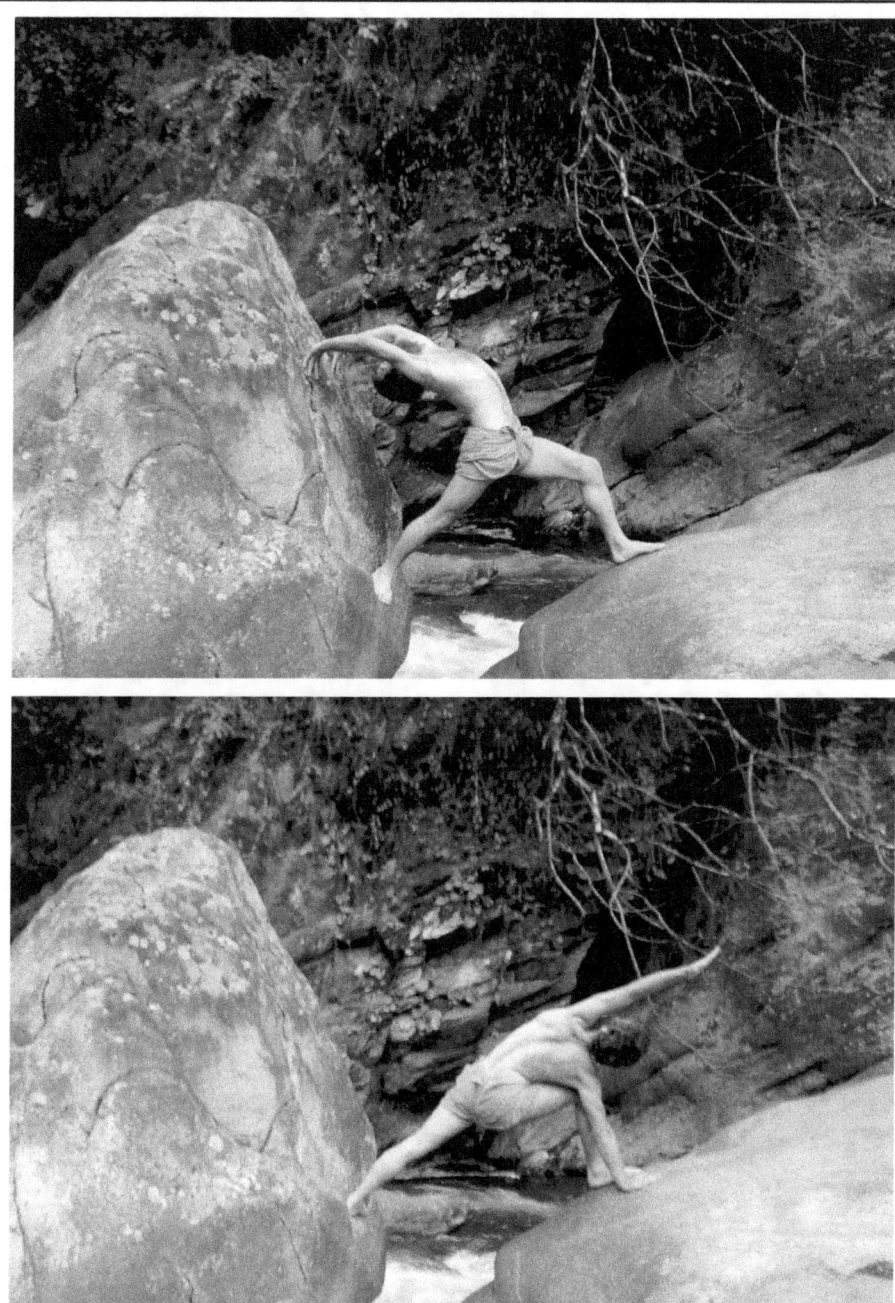

Photos 78-79

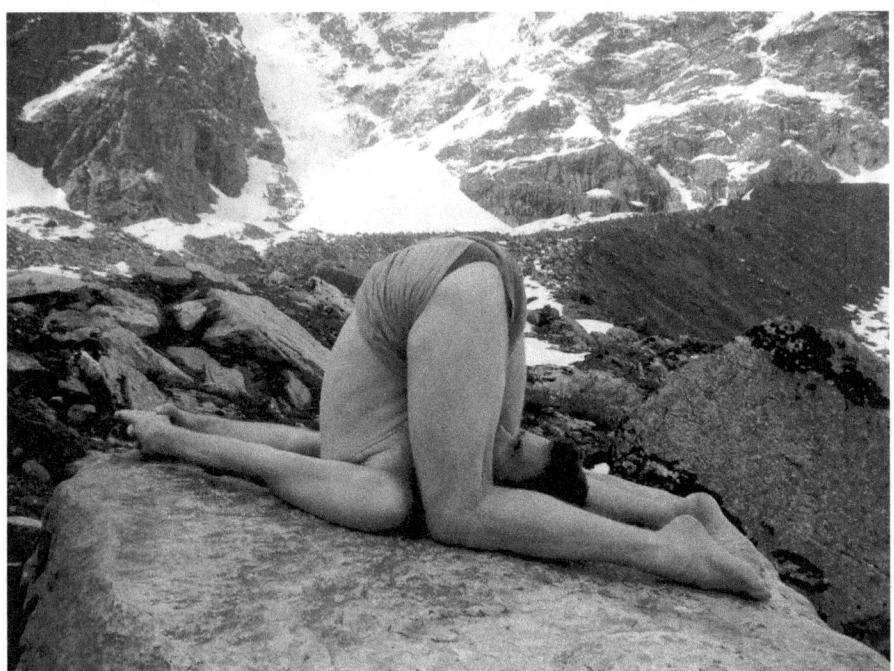

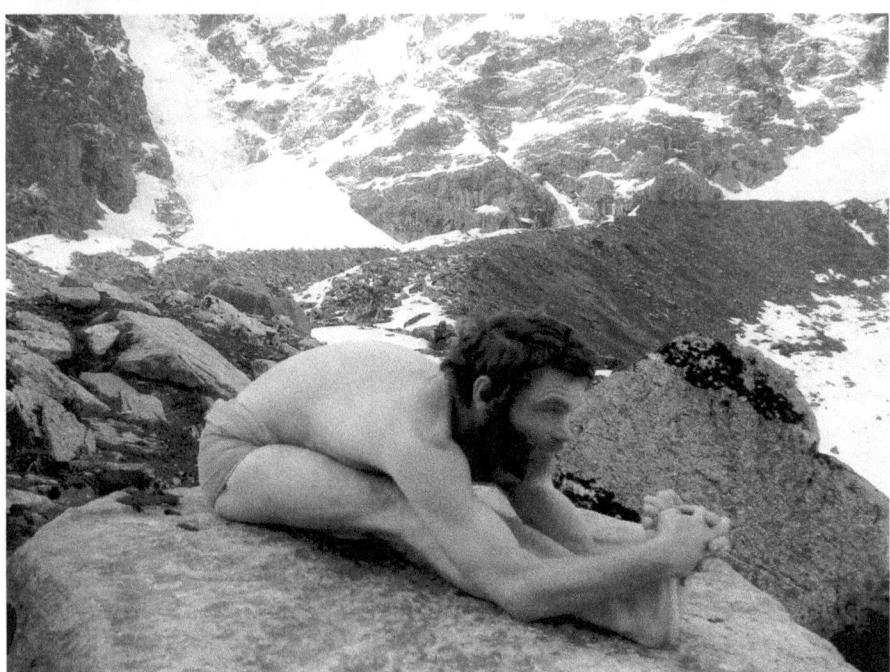

Photos 80(a-b)

Finally, I add an impression from practice of lying asanas on inclined surfaces. Generally we didn't study in this book any postures in lying position, except of some variations with an imaginary 'space inversion', when we tried to master the same form 'lying on the wall'. As well sometimes we added variations with a thrust of feet against the wall. But that's all. However it is quite difficult to find a plane site for practice at an irregular terrain even though you don't strain after improvisations with rocks. That is why lying asanas have to be done on a gradient plane, which keeps tendency to convert into vertical in a particular degree. In that case everything depends on a canting angle and an orientation of your head up or downward... Even a flat slope is able to change performing of the simplest usual asanas largely; and you will find a lot of new in ordinary postures. I give two examples of opposite movement: Karna Pidasana and Paschimottanasana (Photo 80, a-b). In both cases you get possibility to enter deeper in the forms of these asanas.

Nevertheless it is an appropriate time in order to have a strong mind to certain effort to stop, though any interruption is complicated in the middle of improvisation, since universal creative energy is infinite.

Conclusion.
Buddhist 'Wall Vision'

'Yesterday I got freedom…
What will I do with it?'
Vladimir Vysotsky

This is a rhetorical question, since the freedom is doing self-activity… As you know from classical yogic treatises the question about a subject of liberation cannot be answered by an object of liberation. At least, it is true till discrimination between subject and object is essential for the last one. Russian religious philosophy is characterized with a choice between 'freedom from' and 'freedom for'; but this question is not important in Yoga. But because free person himself decides how he wish to define freedom, there is no point for the debate. Although we could offer some content for meditation, which any searcher of liberty can easily perform within the walls of his house.

Everything is good in habitual 'dead-end' where you can feel calm and comfortably, quite in a family way. Indeed 'before wall' is equal to 'behind wall'. However, gradually any walls of themselves fall into decay, if you don't break down or overstep them. Sooner or later we should relinquish metaphors since such a parlance is also bondage of corruption from a province of the processed world. Yogis prefer noble silence, but we would wait a bit before hush, because calm can be correct or wrong too. So, let us repeat the question about freedom: what means the term *mukti* denotative the ultimate limit state of existence. In order to start from something comprehensible and frame proper association, we should look back – at the same wall.

'While you are not able to achieve the freedom of your body, it does not make sense to talk about the freedom of spirit', – in this manner the founder of Iyengar-style cuts off all questions about mukti, and we patiently included some modifications of his techniques into our interaction with the wall. Generally modern Iyengar instructors don't teach meditation at all setting this business as an extremely personal task. However even this sentence about 'freedom of body' absolutely ambiguous. It's obvious after investigation of 'free flow' concept used the above for denotation the very fact that further development is quite necessarily. For example, one reader of my other book *'Hatha Yoga Practice: Disciple among Teachers'* wrote to me by E-mail: 'I tried meditative methods myself, but the appearance of backache and *spontaneously occurring asanas* forced me to give attention to Hatha Yoga".

Let us look at the 'spontaneously occurring asanas' at the angle of 'freedom of body'. Generally speaking, this is far from classical Yoga, where even automatic functions of the body are under control, both inner processes and outer situations become totally conscious. As a result nothing will move (even heart) without the exception of your will. Yogi is always on the top of issues or at least he aspires to full awareness as a distinct from a mystic perception of 'free flow'. At the limit yogi knows beyond all doubt how to input a particular state and how to output one or another state as well as he is able to restore the previous state and proceed it as long as necessarily. Moreover yogi is authentically capable of input and output another person (some disciple) directly to the required state of being, if that person requests him insistently hereof. But emphatically yogi never allows to his body any 'dance improvisation' from the very beginning...

Now let us depart from the ancient raja-Yoga where asanas got the concrete place in the system and refer to the medieval Hatha Yoga where asanas got the practical development. Herein we discover the most interesting remarks about freedom and necessity, expressed in perspective of complete corporal transformation. This body mastering proceeds to the extent of ability to merge body into consciousness and again condensate it at own will in the required form and convenient place. Hatha Yoga schools originated in womb of Tantrism and they irradiated other attitude to human body and any physical existence in a broad manner. Yogis were inspired with a possibility for constitution of transformed body created not from flesh but from immortal substance similar to light. Relaxation and contemplation helped them to exchange their usual rigid corporal shape into self-awareness of *flowing conditions* connected and resonant with the Whole.

Nevertheless Hatha-yogis didn't stand in awe of 'free flow'. The enlightenment in imperishable body supposed namely technical workout of vertical, and we have already started it with the support of the wall. Usually a diffused vital power should be concentrated in the central column and polarized along the middle axis. The mobile pole (Shakti) is located in the base of spine, and the fixed pole (Shiva) is located above the top of head. Asanas are one of preliminary means forcing Shakti's movement *upward* in the direction to Shiva. Some lower types of Samadhi appear in the way, and these states are correlated with *spontaneously occurring images* in form of either ideas or gestures. But an ultimate comprehension identity of subjective and objective reality is Nirvikalpa Samadhi, or free ecstasy without any asanas, images, ideas, etc. So, the spontaneous asanas are nothing more than a peculiar kind of Siddhi that is intermediate forms of Samadhi. In the case if yogi fixes attention on these Siddhi he will stay far from the liberation forever.

The intermediate forms not only have their right for existence, but they are essentially beneficial on certain stages, and my admiration before their manifestation was absent of false in the above chapter on advance. One may make a note of modern phenomena like Tray Yoga style created by Kali Ray (USA) namely on the base of spontaneous movement, or the 'free-flow' theory worked out by Andrey Sidersky (Ukraine) specially for Yoga-masters. It is equally true that there are mystic teachings in Indian tradition where everything arises spontaneously but not only asanas. But they exclude an adjustment for control assumed in Yoga and demand from their adepts another position that is absolute devotion to Supreme Will. Even ancient 'Yoga Sutras' included this alteration, since after a description of technical methods for conscious mastering and achievement of Samadhi Patanjali added: '...otherwise [one gets Mukti] by his love to Ishwara'.

For instance, it is mentioned in a modern confession by Swami Muktananda who practiced Guru Yoga according to Siddha tradition. He remarks how his body performed some asanas and mudras after long-time concentration on guru's image, though he never saw something like that before. However you can find in the same confession about a periodical individual practice in the full isolation also the remarkable difficulties of the following kind. Both Yoga as the path of self-control and mystic devotion to Divine are effective separately, but they block each other. The most dangerous time is the period of emptiness resulting then you loose self-control and at the same time don't get any guidance. But commonly an ambiguous orientation makes such brakes unavoidable. Eventually mysticism and Yoga are compatible but with the reserve.

Indeed we tried to take the next step proceeding from asanas to meditation, but again we turned out to be in well-defined 'dead-end' especially obvious within the framework of Iyengar style. We learned mastering with the wall in its grossest form, and now we came to the wall in its subtler form... So, how to work with the wall blocked your path? There is a legend how Boddhidharma crossed the 'wall' of the Himalayas and came from India to China, where firstly he found himself before 'dead-end'. You see, he needed to establish Chan Buddhism far not in desert, but in the country with high developed culture called Taoism. According to legends he didn't hurry up anywhere but stayed at home quietly and practiced long 'wall vision'. Since then this technique is widely used as the preparing stage for deep meditation.

About the Author

Shanti Nathini (Maria Nikolaeva) - Master of Philosophy; fellow of Indian Academy of Yoga; author of sixty scientific articles and twenty books on traditional cultures and practices (printed in Russia by total run of hundred thousand); constant press correspondent for Russian Yoga magazines and translator of classical spiritual literature into Russian.

She spent five years in India, where she stayed in ashrams and pilgrimed to holy places in high Himalayas; practiced Yoga for eight years with different teachers, completed Asana and Pranayama courses and became certified Yoga teacher; was initiated into ancient orders of Natha Yoga and Kriya Yoga; professed Karma Sannyasa in linage of Bihar School of Yoga.

Studding Chinese culture she learned Ba Gua, Tai Chi, Chi Gong; published her books on Taoism and Feng-shui; got master degree in Japanese Reiki; practiced Vipassana and other Buddhist meditation methods in monasteries of Nepal, Sri Lanka, and Thailand. Now she is traveling in South-East Asia continuing her practice and research.

The Author's Web-Site

http://maria-yoga.narod.ru

Books by Maria Nikolaeva (in Russian)

1. *Modern Schools of Hatha Yoga.* Saint-Petersburg, 2007.

2. *Yoga for Recovery of Sight, or Right Path for Blind Man.* Saint-Petersburg, 2006.

3. *Hatha Yoga Practice: Disciple among Teachers.* Saint-Petersburg, 2004.

4. *Ramana Maharshi: Through Three Deaths.* Saint-Petersburg, 2005; Moscow, 2007.

5. *Swami Vivekananda: High-frequency Vibrations.* Saint-Petersburg, 2005; Moscow, 2007.

6. *Herbs for Yoga: Experiment Adaptation to Temperate Zone.* Moscow, 2006.

7. *Will of Karma: Continuous Reincarnation.* Moscow, 2006.

8. *Beyond Karma: Modern Method.* Saint-Petersburg, 2007.

9. *'Panchatantra': Indian Success Strategy.* Saint-Petersburg, 2005.

10. *'Hitopadesha': Antinomies of Reciprocity.* Saint-Petersburg, 2007.

11. *Female Taoist Practices: Period of Preparation.* Saint-Petersburg, 2006.

12. *Vastu – Indian Feng Shui: Garlands from Mythic Flowers.* Saint-Petersburg, 2004.

13. *Tree Element in City House.* Saint-Petersburg, 2006.

14. *Eco-Design in Chinese Tradition.* Saint-Petersburg, 2007.

15. *Social Logic: We-Concept and Judgment of Our Will.*

Contents